The
SWISS MADE
EGYPTIAN

From Medical Student to Fellowship-Trained Consultant: How to Create Your Medical Career Success Path

Dr. Mohy Taha, MBBCh, MD, FMH

All revenue generated from this book will be donated to the community platform: www.myfellowship.com

#1 International Best Seller
#1 Best Seller in 25 Categories in 5 Countries (USA, Canada, Australia, Germany, UK)

#1 Hot New Release in 34 Categories in 5 Countries (USA, Canada, Australia, Germany, UK)

The Swiss Made Egyptian

From Medical Student to Fellowship-Trained Consultant: How to Create Your Medical Career Success Path

Copyright © 2019 by Dr. Mohy Taha, MBBCh, MD, FMH

Limit of Liability:

Disclaimer:

All revenue generated from this book will be donated to the community platform: *www.myfellowship.com*
Facebook: *https://www.facebook.com/mohy.taha.7*
Twitter: *https://twitter.com/mohy_tah*a
Instagram: *https://www.instagram.com/mohy_taha*
LinkedIn: *https://www.linkedin.com/in/mohy-taha*
Youtube: *https://www.youtube.com/playlist?list=UUZ9Si7ZyEVDBVbqqi8qIu8Q*
Website: *https://mohytaha.com*
Email: *mohy.taha@gmail.com*

1st Edition. 2019
eBOOK ASIN: B08162MBYL (Amazon Kindle)
eBOOK ISBN: (Smashwords)
PAPERBACK ISBN: 9781704416946 (Amazon Print)
PAPERBACK ISBN: 978-1-64633-578-7 (Ingram Spark)
HARDCOVER ISBN: 978-1-64633-586-2 (Ingram Spark)

First Published in 2019 for Mohy Taha by Evolve Global Publishing
PO Box 327 Stanhope Gardens NSW 2768
info@evolveglobalpublishing.com
www.evolveglobalpublishing.com
Book Layout: © 2019 Evolve Global Publishing

TRADEMARKS

The
SWISS MADE
EGYPTIAN

*From Medical Student to Fellowship-Trained
Consultant: How to Create Your Medical Career
Success Path*

Contents

Acknowledgment

They say that behind every successful man, there is a woman. While there are plenty of definitions of "success" which we can agree or disagree with, I was lucky enough to have two women who influenced me the most through my life. I would like to thank my mum (Samia) who is a role model for me working as a doctor (pediatrician), inspiring and supporting me and my brother (Shady) through our lives.

Special thanks to my wife Madleina who I met during medical school in Cairo when I'd just turned 20. She came for a medical clerkship to our university and it was love at first sight which continues to grow with time. We decided to walk through life together with all its ups and downs, fun times and tough times, laugh and cry, here and there. Her continuous support has enriched my life and given me the opportunity to grow my career. Also much love and appreciation to my son (Loay) and my daughter (Safeya) who delight us every day and bear my absences. Moreover, my parents in law (Annelis and Christian) who are always there when we need them.

Many thanks to all my current, previous, and future mentors from around the globe, who believed in me and supported me over the years. They guided me, gave me insights and shared their experience which accelerated my career. Without them I wouldn't be where I am now.

Let's change the world together, "Together, Each, Achieves, More (TEAM)."

About The Author

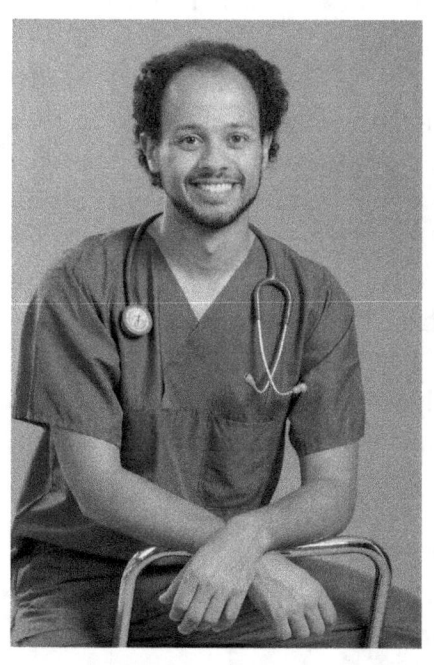

Doctor Mohy Taha, MBBCh, MD, FMH, is a board-certified and fellowship-trained orthopedic surgeon in Basel, Switzerland, with extensive training in shoulder and elbow surgery. He is an author, speaker, and the founder of www.myfellowship.com. The impetus to start MY-FELLOWSHIP stemmed from Dr. Taha's own experiences with medical fellowships. Amassing the knowledge that he has now—through five fellowships and nine observerships completed across Australia, Brazil, Canada, France, Germany, and the USA—as an orthopedic surgeon, specializing in the shoulder and elbow, was an extremely rewarding, but frustrating and complicated process. Dr. Taha thought he was alone in this, until his fellowship in Australia in 2016 where he met other doctors who were dissatisfied with their fellowship process as well. That is when he began to ask—"How can something so crucial to the development of a medical professional be this unorganized and impossible to navigate?"

Coming from Egypt and moving to Switzerland, where Dr. Taha currently works at the Basel University Hospital, meant that he had to learn German from scratch and work harder than most to build his medical career. Essentially, he beat the odds, but that may not be so for other doctors who have the same aptitude as he does, or even more. As a result, Dr. Taha created MY-FELLOWSHIP in collaboration with the VSAO-Basel (Association of Swiss Residents and Consultants) and some fellowship trained consultants to provide all individuals in the medical field equal opportunity to access knowledge, through fellowships and pivotal connections, by linking up information from potential fellows, past fellows, institutions, and sponsors, all of which had previously existed on separate planes without structure.

Over time, with support from the global medical community, Dr. Taha envisions that MY-FELLOWSHIP will grow to become more than just a platform connecting individuals to streamline fellowship application processes; it will evolve into a centralized hub of medical knowledge for all with the help of technology. The goal is not just to make a resounding impact in the lives of doctors/researchers, but to ultimately increase the quality of patient care exponentially. If you would like to know more about how MY-FELLOWSHIP can help your medical career or what you can do to contribute, please visit www.myfellowship.com.

Introduction

Medical Career Success Path

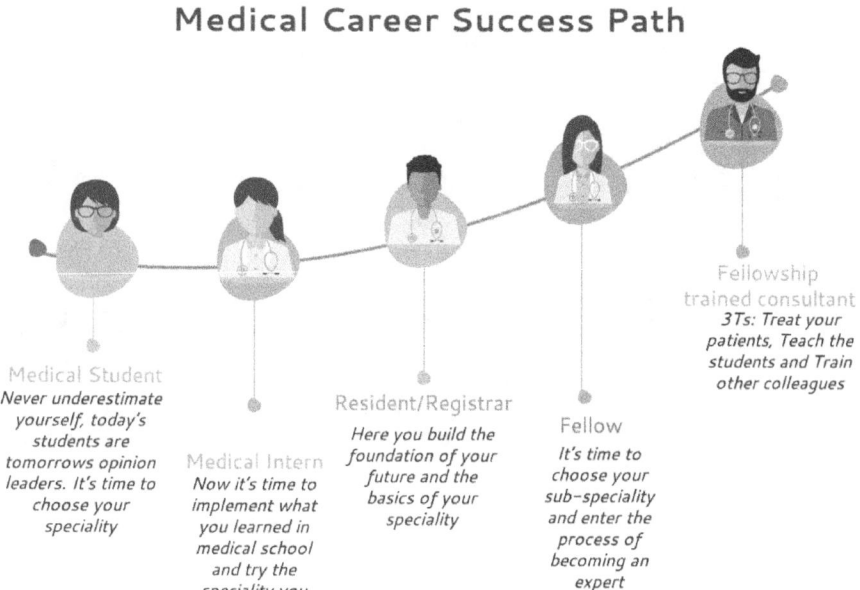

Medical Student
Never underestimate yourself, today's students are tomorrows opinion leaders. It's time to choose your speciality

Medical Intern
Now it's time to implement what you learned in medical school and try the speciality you chose

Resident/Registrar
Here you build the foundation of your future and the basics of your speciality

Fellow
It's time to choose your sub-speciality and enter the process of becoming an expert

Fellowship trained consultant
3Ts: Treat your patients, Teach the students and Train other colleagues

Chapter 1
Your Medical Career Success Path

As a fellowship-trained consultant, with a specialty in orthopedics and traumatology and a subspecialty in the shoulder and elbow, I am traversing the medical career path along with so many others in today's global medical community. As I see it, no matter where we find ourselves on our medical career path—whether an aspiring medical student, a medical student, an intern, a resident/registrar, a prospective fellow, a consultant, or a fellowship-trained consultant—to be the most competent and successful at serving the diverse needs of our patient communities, we should always be striving to learn more, expand our skills, challenge our creativity, and nurture our colleagues in their quests to grow too. If this ethos rings true to you, then you will find The Swiss-Made Egyptian informative and inspiring.

This book tells the story of my medical career success path, one that started in Cairo, Egypt and has taken me to multiple other continents along the way—Europe, Australia, North America, and South America. The Swiss-Made Egyptian tells my story of being born and raised in Egypt, completing four years of medical school in Egypt, moving to Germany for a year, then completing the last two years of medical school in Egypt, and next moving to Switzerland to complete my medical internship and residency with a specialty in orthopedics and traumatology. After that, I completed one and a half years of fellowships in Australia to gain more training in my subspecialty, the elbow and shoulder.

Following that I returned to Switzerland where I now live and practice as a consulting physician, researcher, mentor, and author. And along this already diverse training journey, I traveled to other hospitals around the world—in Brazil, Canada, France, Germany, and the USA—to complete shorter internships, observerships, research experiences, and clerkships to expand my abilities as well.

While my international medical career path might sound rather matter-of-fact and easy to relate to you, the reality is that it was very complex and difficult to pull off. But—most importantly—very worth it. The complexities and difficulties included attaining visas, learning a new language (for me, it was German), transferring credits from one place of learning in one country to another, getting official documents translated and notarized both for foreign universities and governments to clear them, timing everything, figuring out if the people and programs abroad were the right fit for me, and, of course, paying for all of it—both the (often unpaid) training experiences in foreign countries and all the paperwork requirements to be allowed to participate in those experiences. As I wrote, pulling all this off wasn't easy, but it has been, and continues to be (I am still doing international observerships) incredibly rewarding.

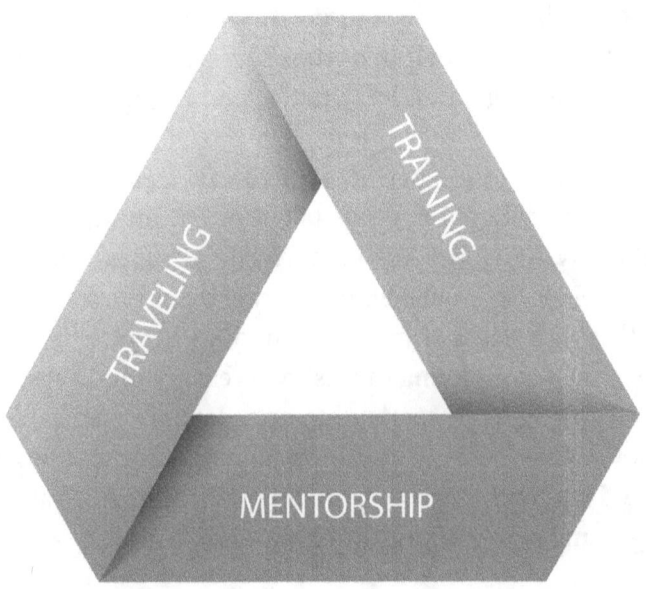

The Rewards: Training, Mentors, and Traveling

I've grouped the benefits of international medical fellowships into three areas, which I call the "fellowship triangle": training, mentors, and traveling. About mentors: through my many international medical training experiences, I've made lasting connections to mentor medical professors and physicians around the world who then have opened their hospitals to me, so I could work with a different patient population, in different hospital conditions, to learn different techniques (often with different technologies) than what I am most accustomed to in my home country. These mentors and the training they made available have diversified my skillset to enhance the capabilities I can offer patients moving forward. Plus, they've challenged my problem-solving capabilities and creativity when it comes to new and challenging cases that I encounter. I am a more capable and innovative consulting physician to my patients and a more practiced guide to medical students studying under me as a result. These connections, with mentors, also result in making available to me more opportunities to conduct research, both clinical and basic, which then further increases my connections, my skills, and my problem-solving abilities.

In addition to the amazing training and mentors these international experiences offer, there's also the travel rewards. For those of you that are travel enthusiasts, as I am, just imagine how amazing it is to get to enhance your medical career and at the same time visit new lands with spectacular landscapes, new cultures and traditions, alluring flora and fauna, plus novel food, art, music, and such. The fellowship triangle offers us a serious win-win-win.

That's why I've written this book—to help others like you, who are somewhere on their medical career paths, to more easily make the leap to international medical training experiences. I'm relating my experiences to show you how valuable it is to your training to put in the effort to engage with international medical fellowships, observerships, and training experiences. I'm hoping that in describing my in-the-trenches medical career path, you'll be seriously moved to keep your head up and seize the international opportunities that come your way, even in the midst of all the demands of medical training.

The MY-FELLOWSHIP Platform

There's another reason I've written this book: to bring awareness to www. myfellowship.com, a platform I've developed in collaboration with the VSAO-Basel (Association of Swiss Residents and Consultants) and some fellowship trained consultantsto to connect prospective medical fellows with fellowship providers and past fellows, so that prospective medical fellows can more easily locate the international fellowships that will make a good fit for their needs, and from there more easily apply and participate in their chosen international medical fellowships. It is a free encyclopedia where doctors/researchers can add a fellowship which they've completed and/or their feedback on it as well. Future fellows can contact previous fellows and fellowship providers regarding a fellowship/ PhD program. Fellowship providers can add their fellowships to the platform and connect to previous and potential fellows. It is a platform where everyone wins.

Benefits for fellowship providers:

- Join MY-FELLOWSHIP's database of worldwide fellowships
- Add, edit, manage, and update your fellowship/s 24/7
- Receive unbiased feedback from previous fellows on the platform (can be deactivated)
- Access and contact doctors and researchers looking for fellowships
- Connect with their previous fellows

Benefits for previous fellows:

- Expand your network to fellowship-trained consulting physicians around the world

- Help fellowship providers and future fellows by providing feedback about any fellowships you've done
- Influence colleagues' careers through the feedback you provide
- Connect to and mentor future fellows

Benefits for future fellows:

- Accelerate your career by accessing these fellowships
- Search and filter one database for fellowship opportunities
- Read feedback before deciding on your fellowship
- Ask previous fellows directly about their experiences
- Apply to MY-FELLOWSHIP for financial assistance to fund your time in fellowship
- Provide feedback upon completing your fellowship
- Stay in touch with your co-fellows
- Add other fellowships you know about

Something I describe in detail in this book is how it took me over a year to determine and apply to the year-long fellowship (it was actually two fellowships) I eventually did in Australia. I describe all the planning and challenges that happened in regard to making this Australian fellowship experience happen. And while this fellowship experience ended up being worth the effort (it gave me the exposure to shoulder and elbow surgeries that I sought to declare that my expertise), it was a lot of effort to organize. While there, I met other medical fellows who put in an equal amount of planning, money, and effort to get to do medical fellowships in Australia, only to find out that the fellowships they eventually engaged with were actually not the best fit for their needs. Apparently, there was some kind of disconnect in what they thought the fellowship would provide them vs. what it actually played out to be like.

To help prospective medical fellows navigate the many obstacles in applying to, and doing, an international fellowship, and to avoid this disconnect—where you work really hard to make a fellowship happen, but in the end, it's not right for your training needs—I was moved to start the MY-FELLOWSHIP platform—www.myfellowship.com in collaboration with the VSAO-Basel (Association of Swiss Residents and Consultants).

MY-FELLOWSHIP connects those looking to do fellowships (prospective fellows) with the people who provide fellowships (mentors) and with those who have done the fellowship before (past fellow mentors). This way, prospective fellows can easily access the parties necessary for providing them the information for making an informed decision on whether or not to apply and/or do a fellowship. As a result, both sides— providers and fellows—will be able to avoid frustration and should be content with the ensuing year of fellowship together. MY-FELLOWSHIP is designed to bridge the gap between prospective fellows, fellowship providers, and previous fellows. It completes the circle.

As I see it, MY-FELLOWSHIP saves prospective fellows heaps of time, heaps of organizing, and heaps of money because it offers prospective fellows valuable firsthand information from people who provide fellowships and people who have already done those fellowships. A prospective fellow can contact these parties from their sofa and ask the many questions they want. When you read this book, you'll not only learn how helpful and amazing international fellowships are, you can expect to learn, too, how www.myfellowship.com can help your medical career and make the application and organizing of an international fellowship much easier.

Ever-Expanding Horizons

As I see it, no matter where we are at in our medical career path, to truly serve patients with the best quality care, we must always be on the lookout for opportunities to grow our skills, increase our expertise, learn new methods and technologies, and connect with medical mentors. So no matter the stage you find yourself in your medical career path, in The Swiss-Made Egyptian I'll share stories to inspire you to seize opportunities to expand your medical horizons, and you'll learn too how the MY-FELLOWSHIP platform is key in helping you locate and seize these opportunities. After all, a medical career path isn't enough. I want you to experience a medical career success path and seizing international medical opportunities is instrumental in bringing in that success element.

The medical field is a global community offering learning possibilities no matter our location. This medical career success path acts as a testament to the awesome opportunities available to those of us in the medical field who are willing to keep our heads up and seize unique opportunities that present themselves, even amidst the challenges of studying medicine. To start that journey, we begin with why: why are you moved to become a consulting physician? We've got to have a deeply rooted why to get us through the many trying times that we'll encounter in pursuing a successful career in medicine.

All revenue generated from this book will be donated to the community platform: www.myfellowship.com

Chapter 2

Your Why

Studying medicine to eventually become a consulting physician—and hopefully to become a fellowship-trained consulting physician— is not for the faint-hearted. It's an arduous and time-consuming trek with many expected challenges, and likely some unexpected ones, along the way. For instance, the applications, the application fees, the competition, the interviews, the hours and hours and hours of study, the plethora of exams, the maze of bureaucratic requirements to get certified in your country, region, state, or municipality, the paperwork, even more fees, the hours and hours of training, the demands of the work itself— this goes on for years and years. It's no wonder that so many aspiring physicians drop out at some point along the way. So many don't make it through the many stages of the medical career path. What makes one person able to hold on and keep going while their close colleague, who is just as smart and energetic, drops out? What is the differentiating factor between those who make it and those who don't?

Whether you are only just applying to medical schools or you've completed residency and are trying to finance a fellowship, no matter where you find yourself in your medical career path, no doubt you have a strong reason for embarking on and doggedly continuing the formidable, long-drawn-out, but ultimately very rewarding journey. Yes, of course, we want to help people, but beyond that, we've got to have a personal and powerful "why" to keep us upright and moving forward.

Your why is likely some key person or transformational experience you encountered in your early life that provides you with more than just the motivation to continue. Your why is planted so firmly and deeply inside you that it erases, and makes inapplicable, the possibility of getting derailed from becoming a physician. It's our why that separates us from our equally smart and good-intentioned colleagues who end up quitting the medical career journey.

As I've already explained, I've endured perhaps more obstacles on my medical career path than the average aspiring physician. And you'll be learning about those later in the book. Here, in this chapter, I'm going to lay out my why that kept me going—and keeps me going—when everything, and I mean everything, seemed determined to thwart me.

I'm sharing my why not just to encourage you to be aware of your why—because I'm sure you already know who or what is the reason behind why you aim to be a physician—but to do much more than that. I want my story to spur you to connect deeply with your own why, to spark you to share the complete story of your own why with anyone and everyone who asks you. By developing that story in detail, connecting with it fully, and then sharing it aloud with others, over and over again, your why will grow in intensity and vitality to keep you traversing the grueling medical career path, even when obstacles are raining down on you. Those who get detoured from the path, they too had a why—but they didn't nurture it. You must nurture your why. I hope my why story helps you to do so.

My Why, My Pioneering Mother

Since I was a child, precision, punctuality, and duteousness were my three trademarks. I didn't need anyone to help me get ready for school in the morning. I made my own sandwiches, and I was out in front of the house at 6:25 am, five minutes before the bus arrived. For anyone who has spent any time around young children, you will realize that this precision at so young an age is really quite unexpected. It is noteworthy, and my mother certainly noted it!

"When you will be a grown-up, you'll be a surgeon," my mother always told me. "You are so precise!"

What a special and joyful woman my mother was! I think there was no other Egyptian woman at that time like her. Her father was from Aswan (Upper Egypt) and moved to Alexandria to work for the minister of education. As her father died when she was in her first year of medical school, she was forced to fight for her position in her family, among her nine brothers and sisters, to finish her education. And she succeeded. She became a doctor and came to specialize in pediatrics. This was a grand achievement for an Egyptian woman growing up in the 1950s.

While my mother is my inspiration for enduring the trials and tribulations of the medical career journey, I should add that the reason I went into orthopedics is a bit different. When I was nine years old, I had knee pain while playing football and tennis. As a result, I visited an orthopedic surgeon. Through his guidance, and the physiotherapy exercises, the pain disappeared. This was my inspiration to become, more specifically, an orthopedic surgeon.

Now, back to my mother!

Don't Follow Sheep

"Don't follow sheep," my mother often told me and my brother. My mother, herself, demonstrated this lesson to us time and time again. My mother always dared to do things that others, particularly Egyptian women, didn't dare do. Her first goal in life was to get her two boys, my older brother, Shady, and me, a good education, like she had received. That's why she sometimes spent a whole year in Saudi Arabia, away from our family, working long hours as a pediatrician in a hospital, to earn enough money to pay for our private school back in Cairo.

My father, a filmmaker, was more conservative and traditional. Investing in education wasn't on his priority list. He saw our schooling as an unnecessary expense. He was the type whose main concern was reducing costs while my mother found culture and supporting other people valuable. On the contrary to my mother, he always tried to stay in his comfort zone, avoiding most challenges.

My mother took us to the opera house, to art exhibitions, and to the movies in Cairo. She was also visionary by investing in real estate. After my parents' were married, she bought an apartment–at a time when nobody thought that it could create big value in the future.

Instead of watching TV, she read a lot of books–books about other cultures and places, like Europe where she dreamed of visiting though she never did until we were grown up. My brother and I weren't allowed to watch TV during the week, only on the weekends, a rule my mother instituted to get us to grow our imaginations in multiple other ways.

Equality

Although we are Muslims, at work, my mother had a lot of close Christian friends, whom she often invited for dinner or whom we visited on weekends. When her Christian friends got married, it was logical that our family went to the ceremony in the church and to their party afterward. Egyptian readers will certainly understand how bold and progressive this was, both at the time and certainly in Egypt today.

My mother grew up with nine siblings, and my father had eleven. My twenty aunts and uncles had about three children each, so that made for about 60 cousins. My parents, Shady, and I spent a lot of time with our extended family. And though some of our uncles and aunts lived in lower-income areas of Cairo, it was not an issue for my mother. We went to their places or invited them to our apartment. My mother didn't discriminate on the basis of social class. Everyone was equal to her. As she often told us, "People are the biggest asset." That's also why it was important to her that Shady and I brought our friends home as often as possible or that we spent time with friends in their homes.

Empowering the New Generation

Another of my mother's dictums was "Empower the new generation." She always believed in my brother and me. While my father was scared that we would do drugs with our friends, my mother let us go and enjoy the experiences of being with others and learning more about life. When my brother studied at university, he worked in companies during the long summer holiday breaks to get to know other people and opinions. I learned from my older brother and my mother how important networks are, so later on, I did the same, working in hospitals during my holiday breaks.

Success Path Signs and Symbols: Your Chapter Map Key

In telling you about my pioneering mother, the why behind my becoming a physician, I want to point out something about the values she espoused:

- Don't follow sheep.
- The greatest value lies in education, arts, culture, and people.
- No matter religion, class, or other differences, all people are equally important.
- Empower the new generation, invest in them, and value them.

Those values act as the foundation for my pursuit of international fellowships. If you share those values, then international fellowships are something you should certainly pursue too. While you'll learn more about this in later chapters, let me briefly outline here what I call the "fellowship triangle." Like a triangle with three sides, fellowships offer us, as fellows, three significant benefits: training, mentorship, and traveling.

- *Fellowship training:* to hone your expertise in your specialty or subspecialty, fellowships can offer you the extra needed training in that particular area that you didn't get as a resident/registrar. You can get important training in other countries whose hospitals, technologies, patient populations, and staff are different than what

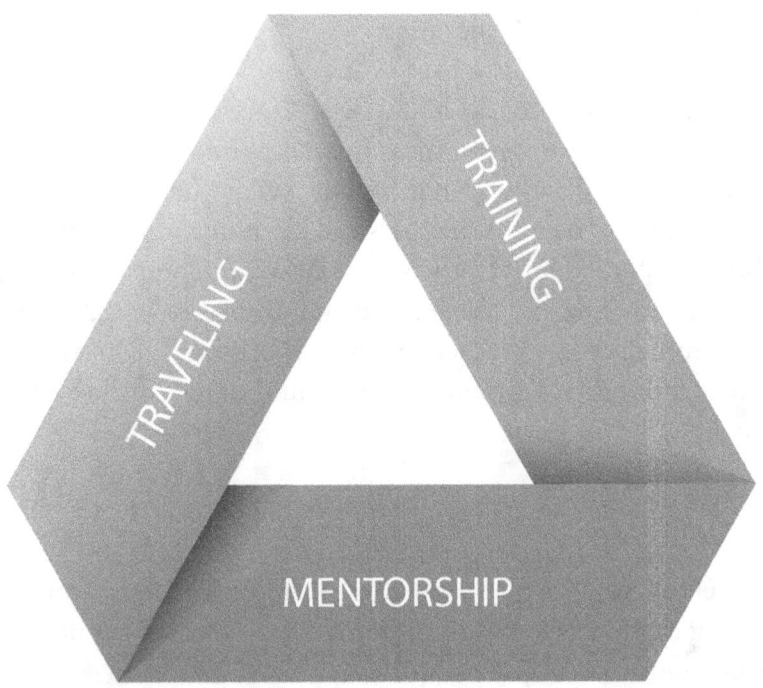

you've experienced in your medical training. These differences allow you to expand your repertoire of skills and abilities.

- *Fellowship mentorship*: fellowships allow you to connect to other experts in your field who will provide you mentorship during the fellowship itself and for years to come. Through this relationship other possibilities can grow, for example, research opportunities, funding opportunities, conferences, and even opportunities for medical students studying under you (this is in the future) to go and do fellowships at the mentor's institution.
- *Fellowship travel*: visiting new regions of the world, to marvel at amazing landscapes, listen to new sounds, eat different and amazing foods, and enjoy novel cultural interactions is the spice of life for many of us. Fellowships allow you to grow your traveling experiences as you enhance your medical abilities.

From the three major benefits of fellowship I outlined above, what I call the fellowship triangle, it is easy to see how my mother's four values readily connect and get played out in the fellowship experience. So, not only is my mother the reason behind my decision to become a doctor, no matter the hardships I encounter along the way, but she is also the reason behind my enthusiasm and serious advocacy for medical fellowships.

The next stop on our medical career success path is a look at mentors. To reach the goals you aim for in your medical career, mentorship is going to be key. The next chapter looks into the important role of mentors.

Chapter 3
Importance of Mentors in life

Through my life I'm always looking for mentors, people who have achieved the goals I have in mind for myself. It is due to my mentors that I've been able to achieve my goals, and it is with their continued support that I aim to continue achieving goals. You've already read about my mother—who set the foundation of mentorship in my life. In the coming chapters, you will read about the other significant mentors in my life, most significant among them (after my mother) include Professor Philip Stahel, Dr. Nikolaus Renner, Professor Laurent Audige, Professor Christian Gerber, and PD (Privat Dozent) Dr. Andreas. In the meantime, in this chapter, I share more of my thoughts on mentorship.

As I see it, mentors help you when you encounter obstacles on your medical career path, and they'll also point out new opportunities. They play pivotal roles in our development as competent and caring physicians, so we should do what we can to nurture the mentor relationships we have in our life and to cultivate new mentor relationships.

While I concentrate in this book, on mentors within the medical field, I should point out that you can have great mentors who are not in the medical field. Friends, family members, teachers, coaches, or even famous people that you've never met but whose books you read—these people can all teach you and guide you. I like to think that I'm providing you a kind of mentorship through this book as well, even if we don't know each other beyond these pages. What I'm pointing out here is that just as I believe you should keep your head up to seize opportunities, beyond simply studying and earning your medical degree, keep your head up as well when it comes to mentors. Someone, who you might initially not expect to be a great guide for you, could actually teach you something insightful.

If you still doubt that mentors could be that important to you in your life, I'm going to lay out what I see as some key benefits to having them.

Key Support in Hard Times

Something we return to, again and again, in this book is the concentrated, dedicated effort it takes to get into medical school and pass through all the stages to emerge as a fellowship-trained consulting physician. I also argue against a tunnel-vision focus on studying, studying, studying during medical school. I want you to broaden your horizons—and to not only do all the studying and passing of tests and do it well—but to add on to that clerkships, internships, observerships, and fellowships with other doctors located in other countries. And to accomplish all that I challenge and urge you to go for, there will be setbacks along the way. You will experience times when you feel overwhelmed and something doesn't go your way—perhaps you don't land that internship at the clinic you wanted or you don't pass a key test. When you encounter the inevitable failures and defeats, this is when you need a mentor. Your mentor—whether in the medical field or outside of it—will listen to you and when you are ready, give you the perspective you need to see the big picture. They will remind you of all your other successes, which will give you the confidence to make it past the temporary defeat or failure.

Recognition of Your True Potential

Similar to what I wrote in the above point, it can be your mentor who recognizes your talents, abilities, and gifts much more so than you do. I remember when I felt buried, utterly defeated by the amount of paperwork I had to get translated and certified from medical school in Egypt in order to possibly (not certainly, but possibly) qualify for continuing my studies in Europe—and there were the costs too. I simply didn't think it was possible. My mother came upon me and I was totally dejected. I distinctly remember her looking me in the eye and telling me, "Son, if there's anyone in the whole world who can make this happen, it is you. This is just jumping through bureaucratic hoops. You've navigated more difficult obstacles. I know you can do this too. Simply be persistent." It was her belief in me at that moment that provided me the energy lift and the confidence I needed. That's what a mentor can do for you too.

A Good, Hard Honest Look

Just as your mentor can provide you that much-needed confidence boost and belief in yourself, they can also set you straight if you get overly confident. It's a careful balance—pursuing a medical career success path that involves more than just the minimum requirements and overextending yourself. Your mentor can help you realign when you get off course—when you take on too much or take on courses, projects, extracurriculars, that really aren't right for you. They can act as a sounding board, helping you to differentiate between projects that will expand your horizons and benefit you versus those that might be interesting but not right for you at a particular time in your medical career path.

A Compassionate Sounding Board

Similar to what I wrote above, there will come times in your medical career path, when you are stuck and not quite sure where to go. This can happen when choosing a specialty or subspecialty, for instance. It can happen when you have to decide whether or which international fellowship you want to pursue. When you have a mentor, your mentor can help you clarify the overall direction you most want to pursue. They can ask you questions or even tell you about times in their lives when they were faced with a similar fork in the road. In this way they can guide you from a place of feeling lost and unsure to a place where you feel more empowered.

That Much-Needed Forward Nudge

None of us wants to make mistakes, not in our professional lives or our personal lives. And sometimes it is our fear of making a mistake that will keep up stuck, which will keep us from not looking for and/or seizing opportunities like international medical training opportunities or research opportunities. We might worry that if we take that on, we will drown in too much work. Too many demands. What's great about a mentor is that they will notice if you're not challenging yourself enough, if you have become a bit entrenched in your comfort zone. Your mentor will give you that nudge to keep your eye on the prize and to go the extra mile. They'll motivate you to take a stab at something new and remind you that they wouldn't suggest it if they didn't believe you couldn't handle it. In this way, your mentor inspires you to be your optimal self.

Your Own Personal Driver

There will be times when you are so focused on the next test, the next class, the next set of certifications to get, that you fail to take into account an opportunity that is in your best interest to pursue. This is when your mentor steps in and takes over the wheel for you. Your mentor becomes the driver and you are the passenger. This could play out in terms of their insistence that you meet with a certain visiting lecturer, that you apply to a certain research grant, or that you forget seeking to do your residency at one hospital and instead applying to the three that your mentor points you too. When you cultivate a strong, lasting relationship with a mentor, you put yourself in a position where you can simply trust in them to guide you to what's best for you. Though you may be skeptical about what I'm saying, there will be times when you'll want to lean into your mentor's recommendations.

Lessons from Their Experience

A great mentor has a wealth of life experiences that you can learn from. And it only makes sense to learn from someone else who has been in a similar position as you and traversed the road to emerge in a better place. For me, personally, I learned much from the experiences of my mentor Professor Christian Gerber (you'll read more about him in chapter 13). Professor Gerber showed me how it was possible to pursue a variety of areas simultaneously and to a high degree: orthopedic surgery, finance, fundraising, and research. His manner of time management and terrific ability to keep organized were notable to me. I should add too that because of his connections and his ability to manage time really well to pursue interests in several areas, I was able to pursue even more opportunities on the international front.

My point: you can learn a lot from the experiences of a mentor.

Heart-Penetrating Q and A

Your mentor is the one who will ask you the big life questions, the questions that get you to engage your heart and soul into your responses. In this way, your mentor helps you to connect with your own heart to figure out the direction you most want to take in terms of your professional and personal life. Although we in the medical field are all about evidence, the more mysterious "heart" of ourselves is incredibly important. Your relationship with your mentor isn't just about filling in the logical blanks, but about connecting to your heart.

Copy and Paste

Neil de Grasse Tyson, Stephen Hawking, Albert Einstein, Marie Curie, Galileo—there are so many astonishing scientists and talented artists, athletes, performers, and activists that people cite as their mentors. Just as someone might follow the career and choices that Neil Armstrong made to become the first person to walk on the moon, you can copy and paste into your life the choices that your mentor made. In a way, they provide a map, a guide, the architectural plans for you to live your life. Of course, you don't have to imitate them in every single way—but there will be times, and in some ways, that you will want to copy their decisions. And it's totally acceptable. That's what mentors are for!

A Leg-Up with Insider Know-How

There have been numerous times that my mentors have been pivotal in providing me that insider knowledge I needed to reconsider a prognosis or even clench a fellowship or research grant. For instance, you will read in this book how I was accepted into two international fellowships in Australia. Pivotal to winning these fellowships was the fact that Professor Christian Gerber, a preeminent orthopedic innovator, served as one of my references. Then take the first clinical research grant that I received. That was due to the support of two of my mentors: Dr. Beate Hansen, the head of the AO Foundation's clinical research department in 2009 as well as Dr. Nikolaus Renner, my supervisor ("boss") during my residency at the surgery department of the Kantonsspital Aarau (2009 to 2011).

These are just a few of the reasons that I can't recommend it enough that you keep a lookout for people who can act as mentors to you, both during your medical studies and beyond. And remember, it takes nurturing and cultivating to make a lasting, impacting mentor-mentee relationship. Invest the time and energy into it as it is highly rewarding, which I hope through this chapter as well as the whole of this book demonstrates to you.

As international fellowships are a main subject of this book, the next chapter tells the story of my first international travel experience. It wasn't medical studies-related, but what happened is informative in terms of determining fellowships that are (and are not) suitable for you.

Medical Student

Medical Career Success Path

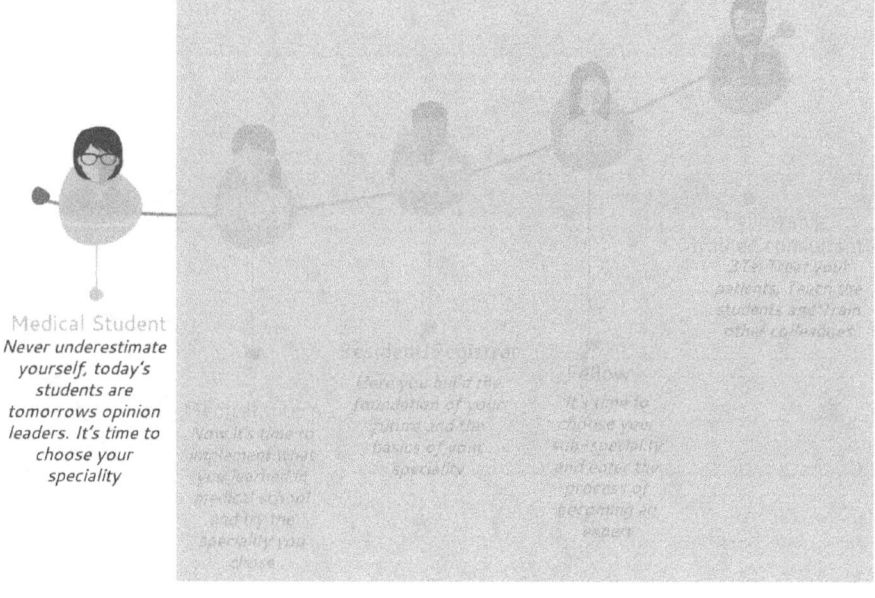

Medical Student
*Never underestimate
yourself, today's
students are
tomorrows opinion
leaders. It's time to
choose your
speciality*

Chapter 4

Look Before You Leap

If you are pursuing the opportunity to do a medical fellowship in another country, do all you can to learn what the real day-to-day life is like there. Cultural differences cannot be underestimated, so you want to do all you can to learn about what's waiting for you there to be sure that it's a good fit for you. Otherwise, you could get frustrated. When you don't do some investigating beforehand, you might not realize until you get there that the different beliefs, norms, habits, practices, and traditions are too frustrating for you to endure for a whole year. Of course, I advocate being open-minded, being open to change and differences, but you should counterbalance that by learning all you can beforehand about the culture and daily life in a place. That way, it better ensures that you won't get overly frustrated or regret your decision to spend a year in a place for a medical fellowship. It's about seeking new learning and adventure that's the right style for you, and maybe even your family's, needs.

Let me give an example from my life that helped me realize that I wouldn't be happy going to just any foreign place to spend a significant length of time to study or train.

Like so many places in the world, in Egypt it is very competitive and very difficult to get a place in medical school. To gain a place you have to be in the top 1% of the class. When I was accepted into medical school, my mother wanted to give me an amazing gift to celebrate all the hard work I'd done to make it there. She'd always told me, "If you get into medical school, I will finance a trip for you."

Because my best friend Hesham had recently moved to the USA with his mother and sister, my mother decided the trip that she would award me with would be to the USA to see my friend. It was my first trip abroad. Growing up in Cairo, it was common to hear about the American dream. We looked at America as a blessed place where everyone could pursue their dreams for success and happiness. Where anyone could get rich. There was always a ton of Egyptians applying for green cards to get a chance to immigrate to the USA. Having heard this my whole life, I figured the USA must be a pretty interesting place, so I was thrilled to get the chance to visit there for six weeks.

Something else to point out is that my plane ticket cost a fortune for my family–nearly as much as a new car. As I've already explained about my mother, she valued education, arts, culture, and people. She valued empowering the new generation, so she saw my trip to visit Hesham in Houston, Texas as an amazing opportunity and more than worth the money.

While I never regretted the opportunity, much to my surprise I found that six weeks was enough time for me in the Houston, Texas area. Hesham was living near Houston, but not in Houston. He lived in a small town called Pflugerville, and the people in his area didn't seem very open-minded. It was a farming community, and it seemed like the young adults our age (around 18 years old) were most interested in farming, music and parties. There wasn't an evident long history in the area or an evident arts scene, stuff I am more into.

I remember thinking to myself, "Maybe if I were here, it would be a decent place to go to medical school. Maybe the hospital system and doctors are good too. But the culture of this rural area, the people, their ways, being out in the country–I don't think it would be a good fit for me if I was told I could come here to study medicine."

That was a big insight for me. I was a young adult, not even 20 years old, and it was my first time abroad. And it taught me to be strategic in my traveling. Even still, it was a great time seeing Hesham.

An interesting side note: not only was that trip my first time abroad, it was my first time in an airplane. I flew from Cairo to New York City, which was about 12 hours. Then New York City to Missouri and finally Missouri to Texas. I took three planes to get there and was in transit or waiting for flights for a total of 24 hours. That, in itself, was a big adventure for me.

I did those same flights in reverse to arrive back in Cairo at the start of September 2001. Only a week later, one of the flights I'd been on, American Airlines flight 11, wwas hijacked (one of the suspects was an Egyptian named Mohamed Atta) and flown into the North Tower of the World Trade Center. I was in a state of shock and horror when I heard that news. A fellow Egyptian, also in the USA, but for the opposite reasons.

And because of that terrorist incident, the fate of all Egyptians, particularly Egyptian males, wanting to travel to the USA and many other countries, was constrained forever. If I'd been in Houston, Texas when the September 11 attacks occurred, I doubt I would've been allowed to leave the USA for months and months due to all the heightened security measures. As a matter of fact, when I was leaving the USA in those airports, I was just a normal guy. Nobody had their eye on me because I was a young Egyptian male. But all that changed so tragically and so instantly on September 11, 2001.

* * *

The takeaway message of this chapter is the importance of investigating the overarching culture of a place before committing to spending a year-long medical fellowship there. To help you do this, use the resources offered on MY-FELLOWSHIP. For instance, www.myfellowship.com allows you to access previous fellows to ask them particular questions about their experience doing a fellowship and living in that place where the fellowship is hosted. You will want to ask them questions about the cultural norms of a place because, as pointed out in this chapter, if you find the culture of a place incredibly disagreeable, it will make fulfilling the year-long fellowship commitment very difficult. This is what I mean when I urge, "Look before you leap!"

While in this chapter I described an international travel experience to a place I didn't find so wonderful, in the next chapter you'll learn about my first short international medical observership experience. You'll learn the ramifications of what happened when I did a short stint at a hospital in Germany, my first time ever in Europe. Don't worry, it was a great experience!

Chapter 5
International Interchange: Opening the First of Many Doors

During medical school it is incredibly common to become single-minded, concentrating only on your studying. It's easy to do because medical school is so demanding with lots of exams, reading, writing, and studying. The danger is pigeonholing yourself where your understanding of medicine and helping people gets too microscopically focused on your books and papers. While many students get by like this, I want to challenge you to be better. To widen your vision. I challenge you to open your mind and seize opportunities that you come across because these opportunities can make you a more innovative, experienced, and compassionate practitioner of medicine. By exposing yourself, you'll not only have more to offer your future patients, you'll have more to offer your colleagues and even the up-and-coming interns and residents that may train under you.

From the book's start, I've advocated the importance of always being open and flexible to potential opportunities. You never know what's going to help you in the future. Doctors and professors you meet in the hallways of your medical school, hospital, or at a short conference could end up becoming key mentors. A flyer posted in the staff room at the hospital could alert you to an opportunity for a life-changing conference, fellowship, or observership.

Be on the lookout. The following is a story from my own life that demonstrates the value of being open and ready to take on opportunities when they come to you.

During my time in medical school, I was walking down the hallway when I noticed a poster for the International Federation for Medical Students' Association (IFMSA), www.ifmsa.org. "Visit us in our office," it read. So I did.

Upon visiting the IFMSA office, I learned that it was an association that facilitated international exchanges of medical students. It served as an exchange platform for medical students from all over the world, to do a medical clerkship in a different country, to experience different training in different hospital conditions. An exchange like this usually lasted for four weeks.

Something else about the IFMSA is that it was completely volunteer run. Its staff was made up of medical students.

As you'll recall, my mother instilled in me an appreciation for other people, places, cultures, arts, and religions. She herself dreamed of going to Europe. Traveling and seeing the world was so important to her that she even made it possible for me to visit my good friend Hesham in the USA even though that trip cost the family a tremendous amount of money. So with this appreciation already strongly built up in me, happening upon the IFMSA was like a dream come true. "What an opportunity you all are giving medical students! Yes, indeed, I want to join!" I thought to myself.

Two months after I joined, the medical student who was the lead volunteer at the organization was stepping down. The reason was that he'd completed medical school and was moving on to do his internship and then residency. Accordingly, he had to move on from the IFMSA as it was run by and for medical students only. This guy asked me if I'd be interested in heading the exchange program at Cairo University, as a local exchange officer (LEO). Why me if I'd only been in the organization a short while? First, I had several years remaining in medical school, which meant that I had several years to devote to volunteering at the IFMSA. Second, I'd gone to elementary school and high school at an international school. That meant that I'd done lots of schooling with a mix of Egyptian kids as well as foreign kids, so I already had a background of being friends with and interacting with lots of foreigners. Thirdly, I'd shown myself to be very energetic, dedicated, and enthusiastic in the short time I'd been with the IFMSA.

I started my position as LEOs at IFMSA in my third year of medical school. It took a whole year to make the arrangements to set up a four-week medical exchange for me in Berlin, Germany at Charité–Universitätsmedizin Berlin (Charity University Hospital), one of the big hospitals there.

In Egypt, there are many Brits, Italians, and Spanish. The reputation of Europe, in Egypt, is that Europe is always cold and raining, Europeans get frustrated by the weather, and that is why so many of them come to Egypt to enjoy the sun. So with this reputation in mind, I went to Germany. And I was very lucky because it was the hottest summer ever, at around 35 degrees Celsius. I even found myself thinking, "I am really enjoying the weather and the scenery here in Europe. I don't know why people complain about it." So that was fabulous.

The cultural experience was eye-opening and invigorating as well. Berlin offered lots of history, lots of culture, phenomenal architecture, and interesting museums. I went through the whole history of Germany and Europe, World War I and World War II. It was a great contrast to being in Texas, where I didn't find things so stimulating. I was profoundly moved by the richness of German and European culture, and the novelty of the food, music, habits, and perspectives there.

As far as the medical learning I was exposed to at the Berlin hospital, it was my first immersion into orthopedics and trauma, which I'd decided to specialize in. I was very fortunate in that there was a great orthopedics and traumatology clinic at the Charité–Universitätsmedizin.

Though I was just a student, shadowing experienced consultants, we had a great relationship. We even exchanged email contact info and stayed in touch. One year later, something I'll share in greater detail in a coming chapter, I ended up returning to them and staying a full year to do my doctoral thesis. That month-long medical exchange is what opened this additional opportunity for me.

As I've been urging you, getting out of your pigeonhole, opening your mind, and traveling allows huge opportunities to become available to you, opportunities you would never have considered otherwise. It's one step that takes you forward to the next opportunity, and from there another opportunity presents itself. Stay open-minded, travel, and get exposed, and you will open yourself to a lot of opportunities.

After finishing this month-long internship, I was lucky enough to attend the IFMSA's yearly international conference. It was in Holland and lasted seven days. At the conference, I met many internationally minded medical students, just like me. Among them was Tanja, the head of the IFMSA in Switzerland. Sixteen years later, in 2019, she and I met again by chance. Though we didn't know it, we'd been working in the same hospital together in Basel, Switzerland. We both met in the emergency department while looking after our patients . That's when I suspected we'd met before. Together we figured out that we'd met at the IFMSA conference in Holland years earlier. Again, you never know what will happen later on in your life, who you will encounter again and where.

After that, I spent a final three weeks traveling–to Austria, the Czech Republic, and Slovakia. In Austria I went to Vienna, the city of music and art. The home city of Beethoven and Mozart, where you can actually visit the latter's house. I vividly recall Vienna's gardens, imperial palaces, and historic and contemporary buildings. In the Czech Republic I visited Prague, one of the most beautiful cities in Eastern Europe. I fell in love with its old city and Charles Bridge as well as its romantic nighttime atmosphere, with lights sparkling off the Vltava River, the longest river in the Czech Republic.

In Slovakia, I visited Eva and her family. I'd met Eva and her family years earlier when they were visiting Hurghada, Egypt, a touristic city on the Red Sea. Her father was a family doctor, and they invited me to visit them when I went to Europe. Her family and friends were very friendly and welcoming. We went hiking at the Tatranská Lomnicky in the High Tatras Mountains. Coming from Egypt, which is pretty flat–plus, it was my first hiking experience–I was totally unprepared, wearing my jogging shoes. Looking at the hiking map we decided to choose the shortest track, not knowing that it was the hardest, as it went up over an altitude of 1,500 meters and down on the other side of the mountain. Although at the end of the day we were completely exhausted, the scenery was breathtaking and the journey was worth it. In a way, this is comparable to the medical student experience in that you know it's going to be a tough mountain climb, but when you do it, it is even more difficult than you'd anticipated, incredibly exhausting, but also breathtaking and so worth it. That's why I'm writing this book, to try to prepare you even more, so you won't give up during the trek and you won't sell yourself and your capabilities short.

You shouldn't ever underestimate yourself as a medical student. Today, you are a student, but tomorrow you will be an intern and then a resident. After tomorrow, you'll be a consultant, and after that you'll be the leader. So, during medical school, be aware of the whole process. Don't think only about now; think about your future. After all, you're studying medicine for a reason: to become a doctor to help people.

While you might work locally, you should think globally. Go abroad. Interchange. Exchange ideas because the future is not only local. When you expose yourself to medical practices in other countries, you see how people practice medicine there, and you can profit from what you learn from them. In turn, when they see how you, in your country or region do things, they can profit from you. So there's that exchange of ideas and research and medical procedures. That's going to accompany you your whole life. Start as a medical student, and communicate with people. Expose yourself, go travel. Even if it's only four weeks in an observership, you will learn a lot.

Keeping in line with this "go global" message, the next chapter details how I was able to go very global and connect with some amazing mentors while unexpectedly stumbling upon love at the same time! Because it's such an unexpected story, I've titled the chapter, "The Crazy Medical Student."

Chapter 6

The Crazy Medical Student

While other medical students might be exhibiting tunnel vision with their books and studies, you already know how much I urge you to take the "both-and" road: yes, you'll study very hard, but you'll counterbalance that with being flexible to new opportunities, people, and places that you come across as well. In the short and long runs, this will only lead you to more options in your study of medicine, and later on, more options and capabilities when you are a practicing consultant. Let's continue our exploration of the doors upon doors that can open to you when you make yourself open and available during your time in medical school—and beyond. We will do this by looking at another event from my life, a surprising "international interchange" that I stumbled upon. One that completely changed my life.

I returned to Cairo from my European trip filled with enthusiasm and backed with new friendships and contacts with German doctors and medical students from all over the world. It made for a powerful way to start my fourth year (out of six) of medical school. It was September 2003.

In counterbalance to the rigors of medical school, I was enjoying the tasks required of me as the volunteer LEO of the IFMSA. Among those tasks was meeting and greeting three European medical students who had just arrived in Cairo to do month-long clerkships.

I went to the downtown Cairo hostel where they were staying to introduce myself and see how they had arrived. There were several students from Europe and among them was Madleina from Switzerland. They were all very nice and excited to be in Cairo for their month-long clerkships that they'd worked so hard to set up.

Madleina and I really clicked, so much so that I acted as her guide the following day, showing her around the medical school. It was "love at first sight," which we tried to resist at the beginning due to the fact that we came from two different worlds, but it was inevitable. Two weeks later, she and I started dating. We were both aware that she only had a month in Cairo, and we were both wondering, "What will become of us after this month? Is this casual dating or serious?" We both felt serious about each other, and we knew that it was incredibly special that we'd found each other.

As my readers can attest, dating and having a relationship at the same time as studying medicine and/or practicing medicine is a tricky thing. There's the long, long study hours and then once the internship, residency, fellowship, and/or consultancy start, those long hours continue. Eighty to 100 hours a week even. Not only are the hours long, they can be long and irregular. Night shifts, weekend shifts, always being on-call. All of this makes dating and growing a relationship tricky. Not all partners can handle it, so you need somebody who has an understanding of, and sympathy for, your working environment. For this reason, it is not uncommon that doctors are often married to other doctors, nurses, or someone on the medical staff.

Madleina and I had completed three years in our respective medical schools, and we both had three years remaining. She was studying in Switzerland, and I in Cairo. How in the world was this going to work out? There was so much going against our relationship. As her mother planned to come and visit her in Cairo at the end of her medical clerkship, I had a chance to meet one of her family members.

When her mother came, not only did she and I hit it off, but my whole family adored Madleina and her mother. Fabulous. Admittedly, I didn't know much of anything about Switzerland. I knew geographically where it was, and I'd heard about Swiss chocolates and Swiss knives. But I had no idea about the day-to-day life of the people, their traditions, style of interacting, values, and all that. But at this point, getting to grow our relationship together was the most important thing, so that's where we were, figuring out how to continue dating internationally.

A Change in Plans

Originally, after my summer clerkship in Berlin, I'd thought I'd return there to pursue more medical study abroad, but my relationship with Madleina changed these plans. We came up with the idea that I'd make plans so that during my next two-week break (in several months' time), I'd be able to go to Switzerland to do a clerkship at the Kantonsspital Aarau and at the same time visit Madleina and her family.

So I made the plans and set up the clerkship. Finally, the time came and I went to Switzerland. I did a clerkship for two weeks at the Kantonsspital Aarau, and I stayed at Madleina's parents house in Aarau. Her parents-Annelis and Christian Ludwig-not only hosted me at their house, but also made me fell very welcomed in their family. Madleina grew up in Aarau, but she was going to medical school at the University of Bern. As Aarau and Bern are only about 80 kilometers apart, we could easily meet each other in the evenings after spending our days in our respective cities.

At the same time that Madleina and I were pursuing our relationship together, additional opportunities opened up to me. I felt I was showered in amazing opportunities. It was a snowball effect of great things happening to me! Let me explain.

Though it's not until after medical school, during an internship or residency, that you have to declare your specialty, I'd been inspired from a much earlier age to want to specialize in orthopedics and traumatology (a story I shared in chapter 2). During the two-week clerkship in Aarau, I met Dr. Nikolaus Renner. I had no idea who he was at the time, except that he was head of the traumatology department. Later, Dr. Renner would become both my boss and an important mentor to me.

Something Dr. Renner said to me that was very interesting and also made a lasting influence on me was this, "Young man, we have problems in the operating theaters with the cleaning staff because they don't speak good German. So if you want to work in the German-speaking part of Switzerland, the first thing you have to do is learn good German." I should add that English was the language I'd been using to do the clerkship, which was fine for two weeks, but German was the working language of the hospital.

In response, I thought, "That's logical. To communicate with doctors, nurses, and patients, which is critical, I would have to speak German. Otherwise, I would have no chance." I took that message. It got saved in the back of my head.

After the two weeks, Madleina and I decided that we wanted to move our relationship forward and stay together. We decided it didn't make sense for her to come to Egypt and finish medical school there because she'd have to learn to speak, read, and write in Arabic. Because I already spoke English, we knew it would be easier for me to learn German and to come and study medicine in Switzerland. So that became the next phase of our plan.

Pre-Plan Planning

In advocating international medical study and exchanges to all medical students, an important point (one we will return to numerous times in this book) is the need to plan well ahead of time for these international opportunities. The reasons for planning a year or two ahead of time are many, among them are whether or not language differences will matter as well as coordinating credit with the registrars of your medical school and the medical school of your new country.

Finding a place to live in the new country and being sure you can meet its costs for regular living—costs for housing, transportation, utilities, food, etc.—can be deal-breaking. For example, the costs of these things in Switzerland are astronomical when compared to Egypt.

In my pre-planning for pursuing my medical studies in Switzerland, I knew that first, I would have to learn German. I returned to Egypt after the clerkship determined to learn German and sort out other administrative matters to be able to transfer to medical school in Switzerland in a year's time. Plus, I was set on successfully completing the rest of my fourth year of medical school in Cairo.

Usually, foreigners in Switzerland cannot study medicine. But because Madleina and I were engaged, they made an exception. The dean of the medical faculty at the University of Bern was very kind to us, saying, "I believe you are the leaders of tomorrow." It sounds like my mother's beliefs as well! So that was very positive and encouraging, something you need when trying to navigate a complicated bureaucracy (and you'll soon see that we needed all the encouragement we could get because a lot of boulders would soon be raining down on our path!).

It was during this pre-planning that I hit the first snag. A very Swiss snag, some might say. The faculty of medicine that examined my medical school certificates to determine how my classes in Egypt qualified me to meet the class requirements for medical school in Switzerland determined that my medical classes and studies were in order. But there was a different sort of issue with my classes. The admissions office of the university told me, "At your high school you studied 11 subjects. But in the Swiss university system, the incoming students have completed 13 subjects in high school. So you're missing two subjects during your high school. If you want to study here in Bern, first you have to complete two more high school classes. It doesn't matter which subjects you do them in, they can be art, literature, or history, anything like that. Do two classes more and then apply."

I said that this snag could be considered very Swiss because there's a stereotype that Swiss Germans are very rule-oriented! But still, seeing as the dean had already made an exception for me (thus "bent" a rule, sort of), you'd think that for this issue, with high school classes, there'd be a way around it. Especially as you'd think it more important that my current medical classes in Cairo be in alignment with the medical school in Switzerland (all of which were determined acceptable)! Again, it's to handle issues like this one that I will urge you over and over again to:

- Plan very early.
- Be persistent because overcoming the inevitable obstacle(s) is worth the effort.
- Be inventive in your strategy for overcoming obstacles.

Expect to see me demonstrating these characteristics both here as well as in later stories I relate in this book! I am simply trying to show you that, yes, it is possible and, yes, it is worth it to pursue international medical (and even personal!) growth experiences!

No matter how much I tried to reason with the university's admissions office, they wouldn't budge on this point about the two high school classes. For me, it wouldn't work to take the two classes, so I had to be inventive and come up with another plan. I thought, "Seeing as I have to learn German before I can join the University of Bern, I could go to Berlin to learn German for a year. At the same time, I can work on my doctoral thesis in the lab at the clinic of the Charité–Universitätsmedizin (Charity University Hospital) where I did my clerkship. After all, I made a great bond with a doctor there, Dr. Philip Stahel, and we've stayed in touch. He encouraged me to return there to continue studying. Then I could apply to finish my medical school in Germany because visiting Madleina would be a lot easier from Berlin than from Cairo."

I went ahead and contacted Dr. Stahel, who, interestingly, was Swiss himself and working in Germany. Dr. Stahel responded enthusiastically, saying, "That would work out very well because, in August, I am starting my own lab. And you can start there as a doctor student." This opened another big door for me!

I started the paperwork to apply to transfer to medical school in Germany. Though the paperwork was similar to the Swiss system's paperwork, the German system accepted my medical school training thus far (and there was no issue with high school classes), they accepted all my preclinical years of classes and agreed I could start with the clinical studies once I began medical school there. That would be after I spent the year learning German and working on my thesis in Dr. Stahel's lab.

I then told my Cairo friends, family, and classmates my plan, "So I've finished the fourth year. I am leaving the university for a year to go to Berlin and study German and do my doctoral thesis. After that, if all goes as planned, I should find a place in med school in Germany and finish my final two years there. If something goes wrong, I could return here. But I have to try this. For me and Madleina to be together, I must learn German, and being in Berlin will make it much easier to keep up our relationship."

My classmates thought I was insane. "You're going to stop for a year to go abroad? You're crazy. You cannot leave medical school. I mean, everybody is fighting for their position. Odds are, for most people that take a year off, they end up not returning. Or, say you do return and you are back in Cairo, you'll be a year behind. The rest of us will have moved on. This is a mistake. You are wasting your time and jeopardizing what you've fought so hard for. Even if it's for love, this isn't the way to do it." Even my father joined these naysayers.

But as I've already told you, my foundation in life and my inspiration for medical training goes back to my mother. Two of her main values bolstered me to follow my plan:

- Don't follow sheep.
- The greatest value lies in education, arts, culture, and people.

Also, my devotedness to Madleina and her unconditional love and continuous support acted as a huge support as well! And my mother herself was on my side, telling me, "You can go on your own path.

You've researched this option. You have somebody to support you there, Dr. Stahel. Go and do it."

While I'd overcome a lot of obstacles to allow myself this German option, more big obstacles popped up in my path. Two biggies (that will likely appear when you pursue international fellowships yourself): money and visa paperwork. To be eligible for a one-year student visa in Germany, before entering Germany, I had to have all the money that I would live on for that year already in a German bank account. That would be about 7,200 Euros total, which was a lot of money. This was because I was Egyptian, not an EU citizen, so there were a lot of hoops to jump through. They wanted to make sure I wasn't going to illegally work in Germany.

The other hurdle was the paperwork. It took five months to get all the paperwork together for the visa. There was the issue of locating and organizing the many paperwork requirements and then getting translations of all of the certificates and getting them officially stamped. Bureaucracy is not something to underestimate. You have to be well-informed because anything that is not exactly the way they want it (even down to the particular wording or placement of a stamp or sticker), can take more months to correct. I wanted to go to Germany in August. And it was already March. I could feel the heat of the deadlines on me.

I didn't have the option of working with an immigration consultant, so I was forced to do everything myself and use any resources I could find. In the end, it was three days before my flight that I finally got my student visa. Talk about nerve-wracking and close!

I arrived in Germany in August 2004 and for the next 12 months (until August 2005) I was working in the research lab and living with Peter and Barbara Jansen. They were my host family and were like parents to me. They were very kind and helpful, and I practiced my German with them. Both of them were pharmacists and friends of Madleina's parents for over 20 years. Every evening after work (from 6 pm to 9 pm) I took a German language course at the Hartnackschule and had exams every month to move on to the next level of German language study. Due to the tightness in my schedule, I was doing my homework on the bus or subway going to and from the German course. It was a busy year.

As you'll read in the next chapter, things stayed busy for me and Madleina as five marriages in one year would keep anyone on their toes!

Chapter 7

One Year, Five Marriages: The Feat of the Lifetime

I was an Egyptian living in Berlin on a student visa, Madleina was in Bern, Switzerland, and we determined, "We want to get married." We would soon find out that this would be a mission nearly impossible. The reason it was nearly impossible is that each country—Egypt, Germany, and Switzerland—doesn't recognize a marriage unless it is certified in its own institution. Each country requires its own certificates and procedures. To make this dream a reality, we'd have to overcome a rather large set of challenges, so to return to the recommendations given in the previous chapter, our three-part mantra was that we must:

- Plan very early.
- Be persistent.
- Be inventive.

As you'll see from the following ludicrous-seeming tale, we drew from that three-part mantra again and again.

Marriage #1 Berlin, Germany

We decided to pursue the most immediate option first. This was how we could be more quickly and officially married, in Germany at least (but it wouldn't be recognized in Egypt or Switzerland).

We went to a mosque in Berlin, and we got married. That's marriage number 1.

Marriage #2 City Hall in Aarau, Switzerland

Next, Switzerland. As I was living in Berlin, I had to go through the Swiss Embassy in Berlin, which gave us a list of documents to submit. Then they dropped the bombshell on us: they wouldn't accept my Egyptian documents directly from me. I couldn't mail or hand-deliver the documents. Instead, all the documents had to be submitted from the relevant institutions in Egypt. But it was more complicated than this. Because I wasn't physically in Egypt, I had to get someone in Egypt to act as my "power of authority" and gather all the documents (as well as the translations, the notary stamps of approval, etc.) on my behalf. Madleina and I determined it could take a year to gather the documents and make the arrangements for our marriage to be official in Switzerland.

So, I had to go to the Egyptian Embassy to give the power of authority to my brother in Egypt because Shady generously agreed to help us with this. Next, because I was in possession of all these official papers, I had to send them back to Egypt to Shady. Then he submitted the documents to the Swiss Embassy in Cairo, which in turn sent the documents to Switzerland to be examined. The Swiss Embassy in Berlin would then call me in to get more certifications, and then they would pass the documents on to the Swiss authorities in Bern where they would be scrutinized. If there was a problem with a document and it didn't pass their standards, they would send it back to Shady in Egypt. He'd have to have the problem fixed. Then the document would have to travel through the same channels to eventually get back to Bern. If there were no problems, each document took around three months to process. Talk about tedious and perhaps even ridiculous!

Take my birth certificate. I sent it to Shady, he had to get it translated, and next that translation had to be certified in Egypt. After that, he had to get a stamp from the Swiss Embassy in Egypt that the translation was correct. Then they would pass it to the Swiss authorities in Bern.

I remember once the Swiss authorities in Bern (immigration office) didn't accept my certified birth certificate and told me, "Your birth certificate is too old." Confused, I asked, "What do you mean 'too old'? I'm born one time. I can't change my birth." Then I realized they meant that its issuing date couldn't be older than six months, so I had to go through all of the process again—send it back to Shady in Egypt, etc. Just sending it to Egypt with a carrier, that allowed you to track it, cost around 30 Euros. It was horrible. In the case of the birth certificate, it was very frustrating because nothing on the certificate was wrong, the translation was great too, it was just that it had been issued more than six months ago.

Finally, when all the documents were approved, the immigration office in Bern contacted Madleina and me to tell us that we had exactly four weeks to get to the city hall in Aarau and sign our Swiss marriage certificate or all of the documents would expire (and we'd have to start again from scratch!). You better believe Madleina and I rearranged our schedules to get there in time! And this was our second marriage.

Marriage #3 Aarau, Switzerland

Madleina and I had already arranged for our friends and families to celebrate our marriage in Aarau, and the date for this celebration ended up falling three weeks after our second marriage at the city hall in Aarau. As is the Egyptian way, a marriage celebration is a time for all family and friends to get together, and this is what we wanted in Switzerland. But realistically, we knew that the plane tickets and visas wouldn't be possible for everyone to swing. We understood that. Two of my close friends had gotten money and all the paperwork together to join our Swiss celebration, but Switzerland wouldn't grant them visas. Why? They were young-adult Egyptian males, which meant to the Swiss officials that they were "high risk." There was too much risk that they would arrive in Switzerland and disappear. So that was a disappointment, but at least some of my family and friends were able to attend.

Marriage #4 Egyptian Embassy, Bern, Switzerland

Next, we wanted our marriage to be recognized in Egypt. Not surprisingly, we learned that Egypt wouldn't accept our official marriages registered with the German and Swiss governments. Egypt wanted its own certification process honored. However, Egypt did make it easier on us, in that we could have the marriage at the Egyptian Embassy in Bern. We were required to take two friends to sign as witnesses as well. So that was our fourth marriage!

Marriage #5 Cairo, Egypt

Our marriage was recognized in three countries! The only thing that remained was a marriage celebration in Egypt so that my many aunts, uncles, cousins, colleagues, and friends could celebrate. We had three months to plan for the festivity. We even decided to invite Madleina's family and friends to come to Cairo for the celebration.

Because we were pretty much masters of logistics by this time (that's meant to be a joke, but perhaps it's also the truth!), we ended up arranging for fourteen of our friends and family members to accompany us on our ten-day honeymoon travels around Egypt. It was a wild and wonderful trip. Really, all five of our marriages were crazy and incredibly satisfying to have pulled off. Finding the love of your life is not always easy, but if you find it, fight for it. Fourteen years later our love still grows, and our son, Loay, is ten years old and our daughter, Safeya, is eight years old.

What I hope is that this story, of the five-marriage feat that Madleina and I managed to pull off with the help of several patient and dedicated supporters (thank you again, Shady!), will give you perspective on the bureaucratic madness that you are navigating (or anticipating navigating) in applying for international medical fellowships. Surely, it won't be as ludicrous, time-consuming, and expensive as these five marriages. Additionally, I hope our story gives you added certainty that if you commit to planning early, being persistent, and being inventive, you can make it happen.

And just like my marriage to Madleina was so worth it, the learning and experience of your medical studies abroad will be too!

That's why MY-FELLOWSHIP is important because you get to contact others who have been there before you and who can support you in the application process. If you would like to know more about how MY-FELLOWSHIP can help your medical career or what you can do to contribute, please visit us at www.myfellowship.com.

From the title of the next chapter, "Failure Is Not an Option," it should be evident that the three-part mantra of "Plan very early. Be persistent. Be inventive" continues as I try to make my medical studies work in conjunction with my international marriage.

Chapter 8

Failure Is Not an Option

In a 2018 visit to the John F. Kennedy Space Center in Florida, I encountered the motto, "Failure is not an option." When I read that motto, something clicked inside me. I had an epiphany: "That's my life motto. From the time I was a small child, all the way to today, that's how I've operated: failure is not an option." This doesn't mean that you never make a mistake. It actually means that you can expect to make plenty of mistakes and encounter plenty of obstacles, some of which you will make on your first try, others of which you will make many (failed) attempts in an effort to surmount them. Even when you've made several tries and failed each time, the point is to keep trying. That's what it means to have this motto: "Failure is not an option." Learning from your own and others' mistakes and experiences is what the smartest people do. And come on—you are in medical school, about to be in medical school, or you graduated medical school, so that puts you among the smartest. Act like it! Be persistent, be inventive, especially when it comes to managing obstacles that you encounter in your quest to become a well-trained, highly-skilled, and thoughtful physician.

As you've likely surmised, in this chapter I'm sharing another story about some serious, backward-pushing obstacles I encountered in my pursuit to study medicine. Let the events of this chapter inspire you to take on the motto, "Failure is not an option," along with me!

That year of the five marriages was also the year I spent in Berlin studying German and also doing doctoral thesis work at Dr. Stahel's lab. The medical school in Frankfurt already agreed to take me in at the end of that year because my transcripts met their requirements. Finally, it was time to start medical school in Germany . . . and here I encountered a stumbling block. Something I certainly hadn't anticipated.

At the start of the semester, the medical school in Frankfurt sent me a letter informing me, "You are now registered in the first semester of study here at the medical school." What? I'd already put in four years of medical study in Cairo and the German authorities recognized two years of my study and I'm supposed to start in year three. So what had happened? Why was I suddenly a first-year med student?

When I contacted the school, they agreed that they recognized those years of study, but they didn't have a position open for me in my year, which in the German system equated to year three (rather than year five in the Egyptian system). As they explained it, in the first two years of medical school, there are 350 positions available. In the third year, because many students drop out or fail out, there are less than 250 positions available. The first priority for those positions are Germans who studied in that university's hospital. The second priority are Germans who studied at a university in another city in Germany who applied to transfer to the medical school in Frankfurt. Priority three, Germans who are studying abroad and want to come back to Germany. Priority four, European Union students from other EU countries who want to study in Germany in this medical program. Finally comes priority number five, foreigners. That's me.

As a result, all the available positions in year 3 were filled by medical students in those higher priority positions. However, I did land a place with the first-years.

When I spoke to the dean, he explained, "No, you don't have to actually attend any of those classes because you have done them before. It isn't necessary for you to do the classes or take the exams.

Instead, see it as an opportunity to be there, connect to others, improve your German, but it won't count toward any of your grades. The reason we've done this is to keep you eligible in the system in case next semester (in six months) a position becomes open for you in your real year of study."

Then he added, "But we don't know. There is no guarantee."

I asked, "What are the odds of there being an opening?"

"We cannot calculate the odds. You just wait and see and maybe."

Right. Okay ... Actually, not okay.

At the time, in that moment, this felt like doomsday news. It was the toughest moment for me in all the challenges of my whole time in medical school. A real gut punch and kick in the face. Imagine my position: getting married (five times) and planning my life for the next several years to stay between Frankfurt and Switzerland, which is a 3.5-hour drive. Getting accepted into German medical school and all my years of study and difficult classes even transferred too. It seemed like a doable, pretty nice next few years. And all the while I'd been working my ass off, doing all of the exams, learning German like crazy, eating German, speaking German, listening German, living with a German family, working in a German lab, trying to German-ize my life. And still, at the end—BOOM!—I am NOT German. And as such . . . no medical school for me. Maybe, just maybe later. Wait and see.

Madleina and I had a big think and a big talk about what I should do. Finally, we decided that I would return to Egypt, finish the two remaining years there, and then do my year of internship in Switzerland. Because Madleina hadn't taken her fifth year off as I'd done while in Germany, she would start her internship a year earlier than me. We decided she could come to Cairo to do some of her internship there in an attempt to allow us more time together during the two years apart.

So, I returned to Egypt, and I started again. Because I'd missed a year, my group had continued on. They were in the sixth year, and I joined a new group in their fifth year. It was a bit disappointing not being with my friends, but I made new friends. I decided to see it as doubling my friends and expanding my network even more within Egypt.

What at first seemed like a catastrophe really wasn't that bad once I was there and doing it again. I knew the language, the system, and I could more quickly study and take exams. I was familiar with how it all worked. Also, the cost of living in Egypt was much less than in Germany. I lived with my family. I already had a car. I wasn't starting from zero.

The two years went fine. Madleina was able to spend six months with me in Egypt as well. She was learning Arabic in her spare time in Egypt, which was a positive experience.

Six months after Madleina returned to Switzerland, I joined her there and I did my year of internship and Madleina started her residency. As the internship happens after medical school, and residency happens next after the medical internship, this is an important time to choose your medical specialty, which is the subject of the next chapter.

Chapter 9

Choosing Your Medical Speciality

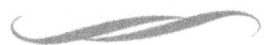

As you might recall from chapter 2, I explained that I chose my medical specialty, orthopedics and traumatology, based on my experience seeking out help from an orthopedic surgeon when I was nine years old. If you haven't had such a defining experience and you are still trying to determine your specialty, in this chapter I'm going to share with you some different questioning techniques and other considerations to help you figure out the medical specialty that's right for you and that you are passionate about.

Some Questions to Ponder

What scientific or clinical areas most interest you?

- Is there a group of diseases that pique your interest? Are there certain kinds of clinical questions that you find very engaging?
- For example, perhaps neurology or neurosurgery most interest you in the area of neuroscience; or anesthesia in the area of pharmacology and physiology.

Surgical, medical, or mixed: what's your preference?

- What do you prefer: a procedure-oriented specialty? A specialty that emphasizes clinical reasoning and patient relationships?

- If it's a surgical preference, consider plastics, neurosurgery, or orthopedics. If it's a medical preference, consider psychiatry, neurology, or internal medicine. If it's a mix, consider anesthesia, EMed, ENT, or OBGYN.

Are there other activities that you want to engage in while on the job?

- You might want to consider a specialty that lets you pursue non-medical areas like policy work, teaching, or research.
- The setting of your practice, as well as the time constraints of your specialty, will determine the options for the other activities that will be available to you. Take some time to notice the activities that physicians in particular specialties do and do not engage in.

Are patient contact and patient continuity important to you?

- Consider the importance of talking to patients and forming relationships with them. Also, determine the type of physical interaction you prefer with patients.
- For long-term relationships with patients, consider internal medicine and family medicine. If you want no patient interaction, consider radiology and pathology. For very brief interaction there's EMed and anesthesiology.

Is there a certain patient population you'd prefer to work with?

- Certain specialties typically handle certain patient populations. Take this into account when choosing your specialty.
- For example, it isn't just children but their concerned parents that pediatricians work with. Oncologists are working with patients who are very ill and vulnerable.

How about the work/life balance you want?

- Do you want weekends off? How many hours per week do you want to work? Are you willing to take calls? What about shift work?

- These specialties offer you more power in determining your working hours: PM&R, radiology, neurology, ophthalmology, pathology, dermatology, and anesthesia.

What kind of money are you looking to make?

- Medical training costs a lot, so it isn't anything to be ashamed of to want to earn a good income to pay back those student loans.
- In general surgeons tend to make more money than other specialties.

Other Options for Determining Your Specialty

Because there's so many medical specialties, make it a priority to explore them in your first few years of medical school. Also, take into account your own personality as well as the kind of lifestyle you want to live: how much time with patients you want, how demanding of a work schedule you want, the kind of patients you want to work with, and the amount of income you want.

Specialty Lectures

Use your first years of medical school to explore various specialties. Because your own class load will be general in these years, you'll have to put in some effort to seek out specialties. One way to do this would be to attend lectures of visiting specialists, particularly if their specialty is one you are already curious about. You can get an idea of the specialty just from hearing them talk. You could also drop into classes specific to particular specialties.

Student Interest Groups

A lot of medical schools have student-led medical specialty groups. Check out your medical school's websites for a list of such groups at your school and attend some of their meetings. For example, emergency medicine, internal medicine, dermatology—if you are curious about those, then meet up with other students who share that same curiosity.

Doing so could give you valuable insight into the specialty.

Conversations with Docs

Talk with doctors you know (or get professors, classmates, etc., to introduce you to doctors) to ask them about their experiences in their specialties. Ask them how they chose their specialty and the pros and cons of it. Be sure to find out what their typical daily routine is like as well. You could even get an introduction to a clinic or hospital that specializes in a field, and spend some time speaking to the doctors there. This way you'd learn both about a specialty and subspecialties within it.

Shadow

If there's a specialty you are particularly interested in, ask a doctor in that specialty if you can shadow them for a day or two. Because it's part of all doctor's jobs to help train up-and-coming doctors, they will likely say yes.

Medical School Career Center

Many medical schools have counselors who are trained to help medical students in your very position: trying to figure out their specialty. The counselor will help you come up with your best options based on your preferences, abilities, and personality. For instance, if you are a patient person with an easy-going nature, they might point you to pediatrics. Take the time to check out your medical school's career center.

Online Assessments

Do internet searches to find online quizzes specifically designed for medical students trying to determine a specialty. The assessment asks questions about your abilities and interests. For example, the Association of American Medical Colleges offers an assessment at this URL: https://www.aamc.org/cim/specialty/. The University of Virginia

School of Medicine offers an assessment at this URL: https://www.med-ed.virginia.edu/specialties/. It is possible that your medical school offers an online assessment as well. Look it up and find out. It could be helpful.

Hours, Stress, and Money

Each specialty has a typical work schedule, amount of stress, and associated income. These vary between specialties. Surgeons tend to make more money than GPs, but they are also under a lot more stress. ER doctors sometimes are on call. Think about these practical factors and what makes sense with your personality and lifestyle goals.

Patient Relationships

Some specialties are all about the procedures and you don't spend much time with the patient. This is true for pathology and radiology. But other specialties require you to build extensive relationships with your patients. This is true of internal medicine and family medicine. Then there's specialties that are a mix of both. For example, an ER doctor is interacting with many patients, but the interactions are short. Again, you should take into account your own personal preferences here to help you narrow your options.

Excellent Skills

In what areas of your classes are you doing particularly well in? Sure, this doesn't necessarily mean you like, say, dissecting—but if you are particularly good at it, you might want to consider an option in surgery.

Residency Time

The time you spend as a resident or registrar depends on the specialty you choose. This can vary from three years to six or more depending on the medical council's regulation. This practical time consideration is something for you to consider.

Your Original Reason

The original reason you decided to pursue a medical career could give you insight into the specialty that makes the most sense for you. If the idea of saving someone's life motivated you, then an urgent care type specialty could make sense for you. If supporting people to achieve longtime good health motivated you, then a GP could be right for you.

Choose Carefully

If you have any say in terms of your clinical rotations, be smart about what you decide. For any specialty you are most interested in, do your best to get placed somewhere that has a good reputation in that area.

Electives and Exchanges

Your elective rotations offer you the chance to really get to know a specialty—so try to apply to them early to land the ones you most want to do. If your medical school doesn't offer elective rotations in the specialty you want to explore, it's possible that another medical school will take you as a visiting student. Perhaps your school offers exchanges with other medical schools as well.

Keep a Journal

While you are doing your rotations, take notes. Record what you like, don't like, the general culture, the patient interactions, and the daily routines. Take note of how you feel by the day's end—frustrated and exhausted? Or satisfied? Notice if you are eager to start work as well. These insights could give you important clues on a specialty that's ideal for you or one that you should avoid. Plus, later on, you can refer back to these journal entries to help you make your decision.

Your Passion

Ultimately, I hope that you choose a specialty that you are passionate about and that you can grow in for decades to come. It's not about making money, following a family tradition, or coming off as prestigious in your community—it's about serving your patients with commitment and passion for decades to come.

Seeing as fellowships offer you the opportunity to hone your training in your specialty or subspecialty, let's turn to MY-FELLOWSHIP in the next chapter.

Chapter 10
Students on MY-FELLOWSHIP

Once you decide on which specialty you want to pursue, or you shortlist a few specialties, visit www.myfellowship.com and connect to some specialists in that field who are from different countries. Ask them about their experience, how their residency was, and if they still like the specialty now that they've been working in it for several years. Find out how others practice the specialty in different countries. This will broaden your spectrum and grow your network. Find a mentor today and down the road, you may end up doing a fellowship or observership with them. MY-FELLOWSHIP offers an incredible opportunity to medical students, residents/registrars, fellows, and consulting physicians to expand and intensify your training while engaging with mentors and travel at the same time.

If you would like to know more about how MY-FELLOWSHIP can help your medical career, or what you can do to contribute, please visit us at www.myfellowship.com.

A MY-FELLOWSHIP Activity for You

Just to show you how powerful the resources are at MY-FELLOWSHIP, here's an exercise for you to engage with it. Go to www.myfellowship. com, and find two mentors in two different countries who are working on projects or who specialize in an area interesting and relevant to you. These would be two experts who could help you to expand your own

 expertise and learn a new technique or engage in a new research project. Go ahead and do this exercise. It'll take you five minutes or less, and it will open the floodgates of your enthusiasm and determination to pursue international fellowships and observerships.

Keeping along the lines of our international theme, in the next chapter you'll read about the international internship opportunity I experienced and how my mentors were key to making the opportunity possible for me.

All revenue generated from this book will be donated to the community platform: www.myfellowship.com

Medical Intern

Medical Career Success Path

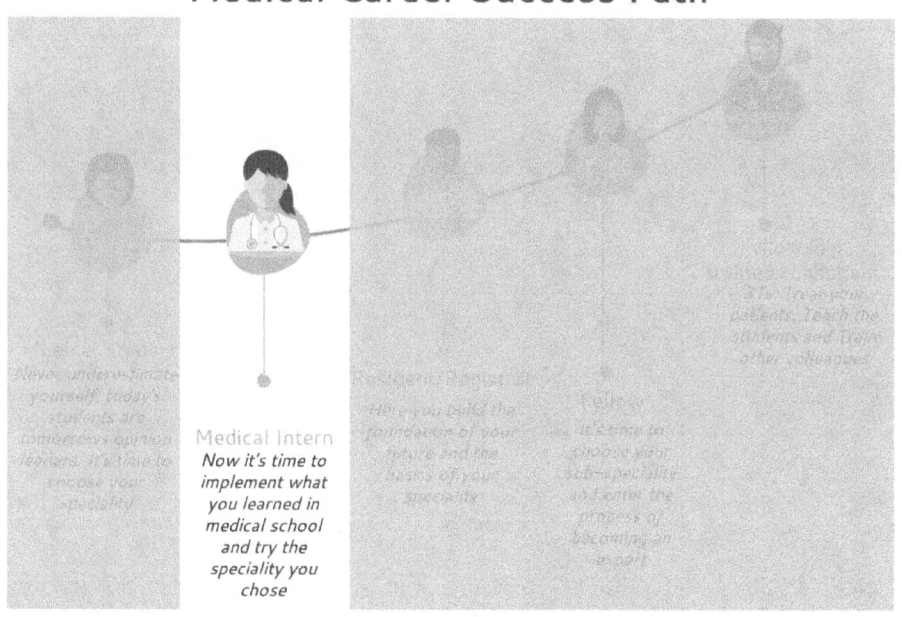

Medical Intern
Now it's time to implement what you learned in medical school and try the speciality you chose

Chapter 11

Incredible International Internship Opportunity

As mentioned, Madleina returned to Switzerland and started her residency as a pediatrician in Kantonsspital Aarau. I was a year behind due to the year I spent in Germany and the decision to finish my 6 years of medical school in Cairo. Because I ended up going to medical school in my home country of Egypt, when I did my year of internship in Switzerland, I saw it as an example of my pursuing an "international" opportunity in my medical studies.

Before describing that year, for readers studying medicine who aren't familiar with the internship stage (as medical education requirements can differ, depending on your jurisdiction), here is Wikipedia's explanation for the "medical internship":

"Medical intern" is a term used in some countries to describe a physician in training who has completed medical school and has a medical degree, but does not yet have a full license to practice medicine unsupervised. Following completion of entry-level training/classroom learning, where you are in classes and labs, many times you are required to undertake a period of supervised practice before full registration is granted. Medical education generally ends with a period of practical training similar to an internship, but the way the overall program of academic and practical medical training is structured differs depending upon the country, as does the terminology used. For example, in some countries this is called an "internship" or "conditional registration." In the UK it's called "foundation."

I started my internship in the general surgery and traumatology department of the Kantonsspital Aarau with Dr. Renner. As I explained in chapter 6, Dr. Renner had been my supervisor during the clerkship I'd done at this hospital a few years earlier. He was the one who had wisely advised me to learn German. Here you go, four years later and I was back, having finished medical school and also having learned German. Admittedly, this internship experience was my first time practicing medicine in the German language. Sure, earlier I'd done clerkships for a few weeks in Switzerland and Germany, but those were conducted in English. Now, I not only had to speak and listen in German, I had to be able to write medical terminology accurately in it too. This was not easy. Franky, it was a big challenge. But the fact that I'd already connected with Dr. Renner and had taken his advice by setting aside a year for intense German-language study meant that I had his full support, which made a difference.

I want to add that my internship experience also placed me in various hospitals over the course of that year. I next was in the ER at the Inselspital Bern. As Bern is situated in the crook of the Aare River, during the summer, after finishing my morning shift from 7 am to 4 pm, I would enjoy a swim in the river. That was always a highlight, swimming in the river and eating some barbecue.

After that, I was back at the Kantonsspital Aarau in pediatrics, where my wife was my boss (yes!). Because we worked in the same hospital, there was a bit of confusion related to our names. As her name is Madleina Taha, or M. Taha, and my name is Mohy Taha, or M. Taha, there were two Dr. M. Tahas. I started getting her letters and she would often get mine. At least it was only two months together at the same hospital!

Next, I was in the OBGYN in the University Hospital of Basel. While I'd never considered a specialty in OBGYN, I ended up really liking some aspects of it. Unlike other specialties, the OBGYN consultant does a lot of work independently. They aren't so dependent on a team. For instance, they do a diagnosis by themselves, they take swabs by themselves, they look at it under the microscope by themselves, and they do the ultrasound by themselves. However, for other procedures, they have a team, like for an operation. To me, it offered the whole package, a good balance of individual and team work. Plus, I got along very well with the other consultants, interns, and residents.

Finally, I returned to Kantonsspital Aarau to do internal medicine. While I wasn't with Dr. Renner or in the surgery department, I enjoyed meeting consultants in the internal medicine department in this same hospital. It was important to meet others outside my department because later, when I was doing residency in this same hospital in the surgical department, I'd need to ask consultants in internal medicine about a surgical patient. It made it easier for me that I had worked with them. I could easily make a call

It was a week before finishing my internship year and internal medicine rotation, that my son Loay was born. That's another important event that happened during this year of internship.

Over the year of internship, there were many challenges. I was working long days, plus reading medical reports from colleagues, and trying to generate my own written recommendations to go with diagnoses. In and of itself this is challenging, but throw in the fact it was all in the German language, and the highly specialized language of medicine and in German—yes, this was one of the more difficult challenges for me.

As already written, I'd been living out the motto of "Failure is not an option" since I was a boy, so there was no way I'd let this challenge defeat me! Not only that, as I've urged you, I kept my head up, so much so that, as mentioned, I landed a position in my upcoming residency with my innovative mentor, Dr. Renner, at Kantonsspital Aarau. Another fabulous opportunity that the inroads I'd forged through the international clerkship and internship with him made possible.

In order for you to land the residency you most want, you must have a stellar CV or otherwise known as resume. The next chapter outlines all you must consider to get your CV into the best shape possible for your residency applications.

Chapter 12

Preparing Your CV

Your curriculum vitae (CV) is incredibly important to get into the internship and residency programs you want. Also, it plays a big factor in winning a place in the fellowships and observerships you will likely apply to. Once you become a fellowship-trained physician, your CV will be instrumental when you apply to join medical teams in clinics, hospitals, and private practices. Remember—your CV needs to be well organized and clear so that it can be read quickly. A great CV is what will open the door for the next step in the process—the interview.

Your CV is essentially a tool that lists out your skills, training, education, and achievements. The information you put on your CV is very important, but you must organize and format that information in a clear, easy-to-follow way so that those reading your CV can quickly understand it. If your CV is cluttered, wordy, illogically organized, long, and not formatted in a standard way, then even if your credentials are superstars, no one will realize it.

A lousy CV isn't necessarily lousy because of the information it gives. It can be lousy because it gives too much information, the sequencing of the information is confusing, and/or the wrong information is highlighted. A CV like that will make you come across as confused, disorganized, and messy—which is everything you don't want to be to get the best jobs and opportunities.

Be sure to read over your CV several times to find any typos, spelling, punctuation, capitalization, or grammatical errors. There are even professional CV editors that you can locate online to help you write your CV. If you can't have a professional help you, then ask a good friend or family member to read it over several times with a fine comb. Tell them specifically what to look out for in their proofreading. Do not skip this step of having an outsider evaluate your CV. The reason is that the care you take in writing your CV will suggest to those reading it—those determining whether or not to interview you for that grant application or that job—the level of care that you will provide as a medical practitioner—and you want that to be the highest level. If you have any proofreading-type errors in your CV, it is likely your whole application will be dismissed.

Here are some standards for formatting your CV:

- Black type (no other colors)
- 10 to 12 point font
- A professional font like Times New Roman or Ariel
- Ample white space

As a bonus with this book, you will receive a CV sample (and much more) by signing up to www.myfellowship.com and contacting Dr. Mohy Taha through the platform.

Sections in Your CV

To make your CV easy to read and well organized, divide it into clear sections that list the various areas of your career and training. Some sections are required while others are optional. Don't try to make the longest CV possible—only include what's current and relevant. If it isn't current or relevant, don't include it.

Required Sections

- Name and contact information, along with your degree and credentials
- Education (presented in reverse order with the most recent first)
- Work history (in reverse order)
- Board certification and other accreditations (with dates of issue, recertification, and expiration)
- Places (countries, regions, states, etc.) in which you hold licenses (include inactive licenses too)
- Military service (if any, in reverse order)
- Awards and honors (if any)

Optional Sections

- Other relevant skills—like languages you speak
- Mentorships
- Publications, research, and presentation

Ideally, your CV should be two to four pages long. If your CV ends up being extraordinarily long, then leave in only what is most impressive in the optional sections. You can even add in a phrase like this, to let reviewers know there's more: "Partial list–full list available on request."

Your Name

Believe it or not, but if your name is spelled unusually or if it isn't immediately obvious on how to pronounce it, those receiving your CV might not want to call you. They might hesitate. As unfair and crazy as it sounds, this is true. They won't want to feel uncomfortable when contacting you. They might just put your CV on the end of the pile and turn to the next one, hoping for an easier-to-pronounce name.

One way to deal with this, if your name falls into this category, is to provide the pronunciation of your name in parenthesis. The phonetical spelling. For instance, take this name: Gregory Afulukwe. Gregory can provide a phonetical spelling of his name to help those reading his CV.

- Afulukwe (pronounced—ah FLEW kway)

Another idea would be to provide a shortened version of your name. This can help patients too. For instance:

- Dr. Ahluwalia (I go by Dr. Alu)

Avoid Gaps

If you have unaccounted periods of time on your resume, your reviewers will notice, particularly when these gaps appear during your education and employment years. If you have any gaps that lasted longer than a month, be ready to address those, explaining what you were doing and how doing that helps you in your current career.

Gaps in your schooling or employment can loom like the Grand Canyon, impossible to ignore or get around. Explain every gap between assignments if longer than a month. If you incurred gaps in your training or schooling, communicate as best you can why they happened, and how they have helped you navigate into the career you've chosen.

Locum Tenens

If you are working "locum tenens," which is the official term for temporarily filling in the work for someone else, still keep your CV up to date. Keep it accurate. After you complete every temporary post, be sure to add it to your resume.

Danger! Avoid!

Don't include any problems you've had on your CV. For instance, don't include any reprimands, suspensions, or loss of privileges on your CV. It's not the right place. Because a cover letter offers you more room to explain yourself, it's the place to explain those difficult issues.

A great CV isn't a guarantee that you'll land a position. Instead, the CV offers you a path to an interview. A path to greater consideration. By avoiding the mistakes and following the best practices, you greatly increase your chances to continue down that path to greater opportunities.

Now that you have the needed information to get your CV properly organized in applying to residency programs and more, the next chapter describes my residency experience, so you can get a good idea of what is in store for you as a resident.

Resident or Registrar

Medical Career Success Path

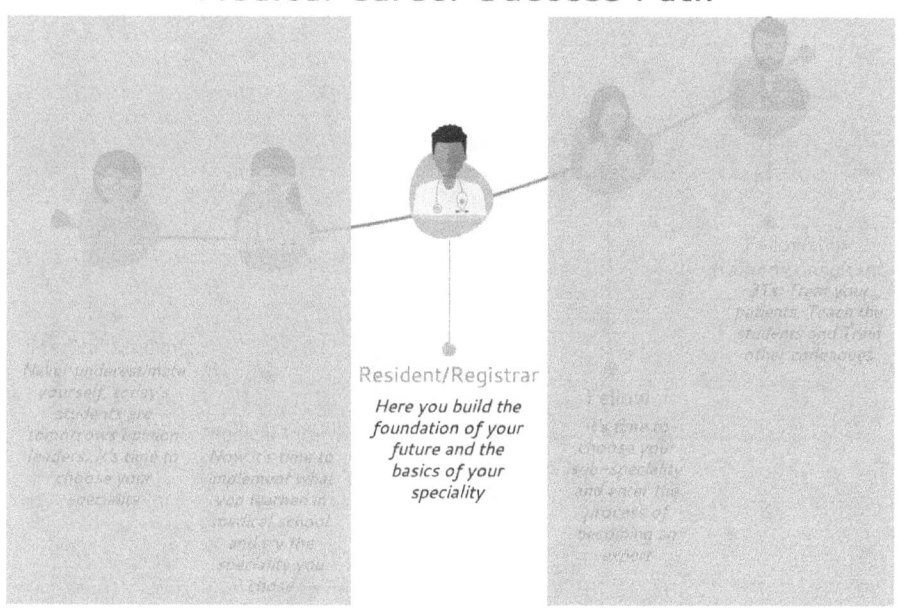

Resident/Registrar

Here you build the foundation of your future and the basics of your speciality

Chapter 13

Overview of My Residency Years

H ere is how Wikipedia explains "residency (medicine)":

Residency or postgraduate training is a stage of graduate medical education. It refers to a qualified physician, podiatrist, dentist, optometrist, veterinarian, or pharmacist [...] who practices medicine, usually in a hospital or clinic, under the direct or indirect supervision of a senior clinician registered in that specialty such as an attending physician or consultant. In many jurisdictions, successful completion of such training is a requirement in order to obtain an unrestricted license to practice medicine, and in particular a license to practice a chosen specialty. An individual engaged in such training may be referred to as a resident, house officer, registrar or trainee depending on the jurisdiction. Residency training may be followed by fellowship or sub-specialty training. Whereas medical school teaches physicians a broad range of medical knowledge, basic clinical skills, and supervised experience practicing medicine in a variety of fields, medical residency gives in-depth training within a specific branch of medicine.

In the Nick of Time

As noted at the end of chapter 11, I was accepted to do my residency in the surgery department of the Kantonsspital Aarau. As I had done my first six years of medical school in Egypt, I had to specifically apply for both my year of internship in Switzerland as well as these years of residency there. Again, I found myself needing to get all of my Egyptian paperwork done to meet the bureaucratic standards to pursue medical practice in the Swiss residency program. Similar to my marriage(s), it was a matter of many official translations, stamps, and government offices with timing a big deal. It seemed that again at the last minute, mid-May, my paperwork was accepted by the Swiss, so I could begin my residency at the start of June as was the plan.

It was 2009, and I was beginning my residency with Dr. Renner in that same department, the surgery department of the Kantonsspital Aarau, that five years earlier (2004) I'd done a short clerkship (and a year earlier, I'd done a few months of internship there). Five years later and I was speaking and writing in German, as he'd recommended so many years earlier, and working with him as my supervisor. Mentorship and international experiences really are glorious!

I spent two years of residency with Dr. Renner (2009 to 2011). Afterward I was two years at Bürgerspital Solothurn (2011 to 2013). The head of the department there was PD (Privat Dozent) Dr. Naeder. Interesting enough his father was also Egyptian, but he himself was born and raised in Switzerland. Nevertheless, we could still share some Arabic words as well as memories about Egypt, the culture, weather, locations, and food from when he visited his relatives in Egypt. After that, I moved to the University Hospital of Zürich (2013 to 2014), where another amazing orthopedic surgeon, Professor Christian Gerber, acted as my supervisor. Professor Gerber has won many awards for his innovative surgical work, he's developed novel surgical procedures, and he makes a point of supporting the academic development of residents like me. He became one of my mentors and helped me tremendously during my residency time with him and beyond. The last year of residency (2015) was back to Aarau but in the department of orthopedic surgery under the supervision of PD Dr. Karim Eid. More interesting is that Dr. Eid's father was also Egyptian and similar to Dr. Helmy, Dr. Eid was also born and raised in Switzerland.

Professor Gerber was not only the head of the hospital department, but he was also the medical director and the CEO of Balgrist University Hospital in Zürich. He is multi-talented and able to pursue a variety of projects simultaneously. He excels in all he does, even in the budgeting and business aspects. During the time I was with him, he was building the Balgrist's campus into a huge center for both basic research and clinical research. He was a very good fundraiser, raising millions from private investors, and had many connections. For me, he demonstrated how to pursue interests in different disciplines to a high degree: orthopedic surgery, finance, fundraising, and research. His manner of time management and terrific organization were notable to me.

Because of his connections and his ability to manage time really well so as to pursue interests in several areas, I was able to pursue even more opportunities on the international front. In chapter 15, I'll share a major international endeavor I pursued that was inspired by my own zest for travel but also by the possibilities Professor Gerber inspired me to engage with, no matter how busy my current schedule might seem. In the next chapter, I'll share another opportunity that my other mentor Dr. Renner helped me seize. Chapters 14 and 15 (and beyond) continue this theme of the importance of mentors and of engaging with possibilities even in the midst of your super busy, super hectic medical education journey!

For more tips for residency, visit www.myfellowship.com and once you register, please contact Dr. Mohy Taha through the platform to receive the tips and much more bonus material.

Chapter 14

Davos: Gateway to So Much More

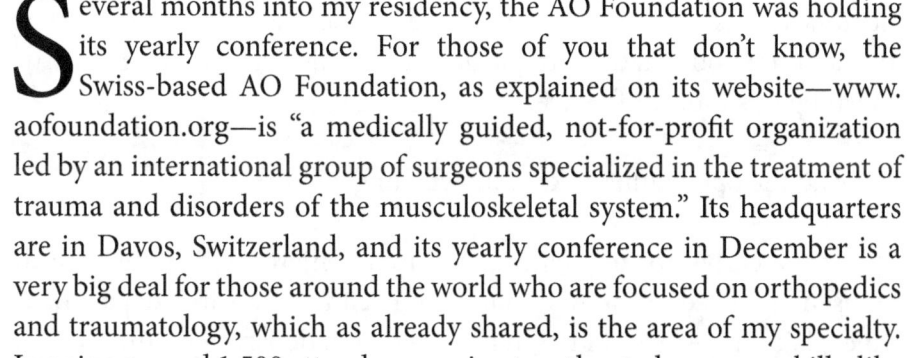

S everal months into my residency, the AO Foundation was holding its yearly conference. For those of you that don't know, the Swiss-based AO Foundation, as explained on its website—www. aofoundation.org—is "a medically guided, not-for-profit organization led by an international group of surgeons specialized in the treatment of trauma and disorders of the musculoskeletal system." Its headquarters are in Davos, Switzerland, and its yearly conference in December is a very big deal for those around the world who are focused on orthopedics and traumatology, which as already shared, is the area of my specialty. Imagine around 1,500 attendees coming together to learn new skills, like how screws and plates work to fix fractures, and all the while expanding their contacts and networks. As an aside, let me add that when you complete medical school and go into your internship and later residency in orthopedics and traumatology, it is a huge milestone when you finally learn how to fix fractures. That's when you move out of the theory and reading, and proceed into practical, hands-on skills. And at this conference, there was a lot of learning about innovations in practicing hands-on skills, so it's very exciting for those of us in the speciality.

I was fortunate in that my boss and mentor at the hospital, Dr. Nikolaus Renner, was working a lot with the foundation. As a result, he understood the value of the conference and agreed to cover the costs and provide me the time away to attend. But this isn't where my seizing of opportunities ended!

While there (December 2009), I was fortunate enough to learn about an offshoot course that was being held onsite at the conference. This offshoot course was called "A Road-Map to Clinical Research," and it was held in the early morning, around 6:30 am, before the primary conference started. Though I'd done basic research in Dr. Stahel's lab in Berlin, I'd never done clinical research. As explained on the site www.earn-eye.eu, "Clinical research refers to all research carried out on humans (healthy or sick people). It focuses on improving knowledge of diseases, developing diagnostic methods and new treatments or medical devices to ensure better patient care." What an opportunity! I'd never done research involving humans, only studies involving animal organisms. So, even though it meant getting up early after a long night out socializing with established, leading, and/or up-and-coming medical doctors I'd just met at the conference, I knew it was worth pushing through my body's fatigue to participate in this clinical research early-morning offshoot conference.

And the opportunities kept snowballing!

At the early-morning clinical research conference, I met Dr. Beate Hansen, the head of the AO Foundation's clinical research department. To explain: the AO Foundation has a research department, the AOCID in Dubendorf, Switzerland, which runs all of their multinational, clinical research studies as well as basic research studies. Dr. Hansen informed those of us participating in the early-morning conference that her department offered a fellowship program for clinical research. The fellowship consisted of three months with top clinical research doctors who were conducting clinical research studies worldwide for multi-center studies. Participating fellows would learn from them about conducting multi-center research and clinical research studies, as well as how to get medical devices, international recognition, and how to navigate the many regulations. They also would help fellows with statistical analysis and getting fellows' studies published. I was super excited about this fellowship opportunity.

Dr. Hansen explained that to apply, you have to present your own project, an original issue you'd like to do clinical research on. I was motivated to participate, but I didn't immediately have an issue in orthopedics and traumatology that I already knew I wanted to investigate.

After the fabulous AO Foundation conference, I returned to the hospital and consulted with Dr. Renner. I told him about the three-month clinical research fellowship that Dr. Hansen described and how I'd like to do it. He pointed out exactly what Dr. Hansen had said, "Mohy, you'll have to come up with a study idea. That's what you need to make it happen."

Two days later the idea came to me when I was working with the emergency room doctors and seeing some elderly patients with fractures of the neck of femur that we were treating without operations. I reported the following to Dr. Renner, "I know we treat many fractures with an operation, so how are these people leaving the ER without an operation? Will they need an operation in the future? Or do they somehow never need operations?"

In response, Dr. Renner said, "That's a good question. We don't know because we don't follow them that long. They come once when they have the fracture, and they come again six weeks later, and that's it."

"This is what I'd like to do a study on," I told him.

This is how my idea for a study came about. I would follow up on these fracture patients and see if they truly proceeded well without operations or if they ended up needing operations later. From there, I applied for the fellowship, and I got accepted. The fellowship, which I did two years into my residency (2011), was yet another turning point in my career, learning about clinical research and conducting clinical studies with the world's top orthopedics and traumatology medical researchers at the AOCID. Another highlight in April 2011 was the birth of our daughter "Safeya" who delight us every day.

My mentor during the fellowship was Professor Laurent Audigé who was originally a vet and epidemiologist. He has huge experience in clinical statistics in orthopedic surgery. One of the major lessons I learned from him was "Don't calculate it, just program it" referring to data analysis of the research projects. At that time he introduced me to PD Dr. Andreas Mueller who is currently the head of the shoulder and elbow unit and my current mentor at Basel University Hospital. Although my fellowship was in 2011, I'm still in contact with Professor Audigé, and we collaborate on multiple research projects.

If you'd like to check out the study, here's the reference information to help you locate it:

Mohy E. Taha, Laurent Audigé, Gregor Siegel, and Nikolaus Renner, "Factors Predicting Secondary Displacement After Non-operative Treatment of Undisplaced Femoral Neck Fractures," Archives of Orthopaedic and Trauma Surgery 135, no. 2 (February 2015): 243—249, doi: 10.1007/s00402-014-2139-9, https://www.ncbi.nlm.nih.gov/pubmed/25550094.

The big takeaway I'm hoping to impart to you is one I've iterated several times already, but as you can see, it can't be iterated enough: even in the midst of all the demands of your medical training, keep your head up and on the lookout for opportunities, which may come in the form of new mentors, events, or paths of study. You never know when you will come across a remarkable opportunity. Always be open and flexible, for you never know what's going to help you in the future. This is the very subject of the next chapter: being open, flexible, and enthusiastic to pursue amazing opportunities.

Chapter 15

Why a Fellowship?

Plenty of graduating residents apply for a fellowship and the demand is increasing. There are plenty of reasons why residents choose to do a fellowship. Here I explore some of these reasons with you.

Expansion of Knowledge and Research Opportunities

The subspecialization is a response to the daily increasing amount of knowledge, which requires that trainees gain command of a far greater body of knowledge than in the past. There has also been a shift in how disease processes are treated. There are plenty of research fields evolving every day.

Advances in Technology

Also, advances in technology require surgeons to learn entirely new sets of skills than open surgery. The introduction of arthroscopy, laparoscopic, and thoracoscopic surgery demands that trainees obtain a new skill set during their years of residency training. The introduction of minimal invasive techniques requires more training. Moreover, robots are being using more frequently, not to forget that 3D planning tools, simulators, and augmented reality are all becoming part of our everyday tools.

Reduction in Training Hours

Limitations placed on resident work hours directly affect current residency training. The goals of duty-hour restrictions were to improve patient safety, resident education, and overall resident wellbeing. On the other side, more diseases and conditions are treated nonoperatively than in the past due to improvements in medication. This means that the volume of cases with which residents graduate is lower than what is deemed necessary to provide confidence in independent practice.

Insurance and Malpractice

The decreased tolerance to complications, along with increased legislation and lawsuits against physicians, requires the presence of a senior supervision during each operation. This reduces the independence of residents.

Perception That Subspecialization Improves Patient Care

The public perception that better care can be provided by specialists, such as those with fellowship training, has also made subspecialization more attractive. Advertising and market forces attempt to draw patients to physicians who have subspecialty training. There have been attempts to regionalize complex surgical cases, bringing patients to centers with higher volumes and fellowship-trained specialists. For instance, in the United States, there are more than 20 recognized specialty fellowships of surgery.

How Can a Fellowship Help?

Fellowships enhance skills, with additional training providing the graduating resident with an opportunity to master surgical, clinical, interventional, or research skills as well as gain confidence, progressive autonomy, and receive further mentorship.

The fellowship training also helps trainees to obtain desired positions and facilitates the transition from formal training to independent practice. It allows the resident to tailor their training to match their personal interests and future practice goals.

In Switzerland especially, there's a high physician density. While this might be great for Swiss citizens, for surgeons in residency, as I was, it made it difficult to get the hands-on surgery training that I needed. I imagine many of my medical student, resident, fellow, and consulting physician readers will sympathize with this challenge. The solution I found for myself, and that I offer readers, is the international fellowship. Through MY-FELLOWSHIP, medical students, residents, and fellows will have a much easier time managing the logistics of finding the best fit for an international fellowship than I did. Ultimately my international fellowship experience proved fruitful though logistically it was expensive and complex to pull off. Let's look more into the international fellowship as a solution to the physician density challenge.

It was 2013 and I was four years into my six-year residency program and I began the planning to make the 2016 fellowship in Australia possible.

Planning out a fellowship is a big deal. There are a lot of complexities to it, in terms of locating the right fit of medical work abroad, the financials, the paperwork around certifications and visas, and the daily living arrangements, especially if your family accompanies you. The reason I developed MY-FELLOWSHIP is so that up-and-coming fellowship seekers will have an easy resource to learn about all the complexities of pulling off an international fellowship upfront in order to have an easier time making this important exchange happen. Keep that in mind as you read about the complexities I had to maneuver through in the coming chapters.

All revenue generated from this book will be donated to the community platform:www.myfellowship.com

Chapter 16

Down Under Is the Place to Go

Which Fellowship(s)?

As noted, it was 2013 when I decided Australia seemed like a great place for me to do a year of fellowship in 2016, and I started the planning involved to make this happen. My first question to answer: which fellowship(s) in Australia would be the right fit for me?

To find options, I checked the website of the Orthopaedic Association for available fellowships in Australia. The website gave me a list of about 170 opportunities. From there, to narrow it down I applied some filters, starting with location. "Hmm, three places my family and I would like to go to in Australia are . . . Sydney, Brisbane, and Melbourne." As I already knew my subspecialty, the shoulder and elbow, I then had plenty of filters to apply. I looked for shoulder and elbow fellowships in those three cities. I pressed a button, and the list of 170 narrowed to 26. That was still a lot, but much more manageable.

My next move was to contact each of the centers associated with the 26 fellowships to inquire about the possibility of an interview. Out of these 26, I had 13 replies for interviews. Great!

Information Gathering: Current Fellows

I also asked the 13 centers about the possibility of speaking to their current fellows. This is very important to do in order to avoid frustration later on when you do a particular fellowship. Contact the fellows who are working there currently and ask them the questions you want answered so that you are able to gather complete information about the experience.

By speaking to the current fellows and asking a ton of questions, I was doing all I could to avoid going on a yearlong "blind date," so to speak. I mean, you don't even go to a three-course meal with somebody you don't know. Instead, you go out for a drink first and then decide if you're going to go for a whole dinner. For me, I was thinking, "I'm looking to spend a year with these guys, so I better learn all I can about how they work, how the Australian medical system works, and get that basic information to better ensure I choose the fellowship that is right for me and my needs. Otherwise, it could be a long year and even put the start of my career in jeopardy."

Interview Whirlwind

I arranged 13 interviews at centers in Sydney, Brisbane, and Melbourne. My family and I decided to make a holiday out of it. We'd spend four weeks total in Australia, and I would split my time between my family and work. That meant traveling and holiday experiences, and also long days of interviews. We spent one week in Sydney, and I had four interviews over two days during that week. We drove north, following the coast and sightseeing, to make it to Brisbane where I had three interviews. Then I flew to Melbourne where I also had more interviews.

Visiting the centers and the cities where they were located to meet the mentor doctors and current fellows and learn as much information as I could was crucial in helping me make the most informed decision possible about which fellowships I should apply to. That's the way I did it.

Pulling off this interview-vacation trip in itself was massive. My wife and I both took off four full weeks of unpaid leave. The journey costed more than $10,000. It took around six months to organize everything.

Fellowship Offers

In the end I got accepted for a fellowship with the Sydney Shoulder Research Institute (SSRI). I should add that Professor Christian Gerber, my mentor and supervisor during my residency years in Zurich, wrote me letters of recommendation, which were instrumental in getting me this, and a second, fellowship offer. Because of his worldwide fame and his support of me, I came across as very valuable. I'm pointing this out as just another way to urge you to take the time and effort to form strong connections with your supervising professors, and really with pretty much everyone you encounter in your medical education journey. We rising doctors and established doctors can be great resources for one another!

About the fellowship offer: the SSRI offered me a fellowship with a one-to-five ratio of doing the operations vs. assisting in the operations. During my fellowship in Sydney, I got accepted to do a fellowship with the Brisbane Hand and Upper Limb Research Institute (so a second fellowship), and because it would take place mainly in a public hospital, I would be in the position of doing many elbow and shoulder operations. Fellowship in public hospitals allows you to do a lot more (as opposed to simply watching or assisting). In private settings, there is less doing and more assisting. As I see it, it's ideal to be able to do a mixture of work in both public and private environments. In private hospitals, through assisting there's a lot of learning, and then going to the public hospital you get the opportunity to apply that learning. I saw the mixture of situations the fellowships offered me as great for the subspecialty exposure I was looking for.

MY-FELLOWSHIP: Completing the Circle

The aim of MY-FELLOWSHIP is to provide massive assistance so that aspiring fellows don't have to figure out each and every obstacle on their own, as I did. On the MY-FELLOWSHIP platform you can directly filter all fellowships according to location, specialty, and subspecialty. You can read feedback from past fellows who did particular fellowships, and you can contact them directly to ask specific questions. As I mentioned already, getting information directly from fellows who have actually done the fellowship(s) you are most interested in is incredibly helpful.

Later on, during my fellowship in Australia, I met several fellows who were frustrated with their fellowship experience. They said it wasn't what they'd expected, "It's not what I was looking for, but when I applied, it seemed perfect." I wondered if the problem wasn't the fellowship they were doing, but that they hadn't had the complete information to make an informed decision. It was my interactions with these dissatisfied fellows that sparked the idea in me that there was a need for a platform to connect those looking to do fellowships (prospective fellows) with those who provide fellowships (your mentors) and with those who have done the fellowships before (past fellows). This way, prospective fellows can easily access the parties necessary for providing them the information for making an informed decision. As a result, both sides will be able to avoid frustration. Think about the fellowship provider, the mentor: when that mentor has a frustrated mentee (fellow), then the mentee isn't providing the quality of work or motivation expected and needed. MY-FELLOWSHIP is designed to bridge the gap between fellowship providers, future fellows, and previous fellows. It completes the circle.

As I see it, MY-FELLOWSHIP saves prospective fellows heaps of time, heaps of organizing, and heaps of money because of the firsthand information it provides from people who provide fellowships and people who have already done them. A prospective fellow can contact these parties from their sofa and ask the many questions they need answered. If you would like to know more about how MY-FELLOWSHIP can help your medical career or what you can do to contribute, please visit us at www.myfellowship.com.

Before detailing my year-long Australian fellowship, the coming chapters are dedicated to advice on how to survive residency.

Chapter 17

Advice on Residency Interviews

When interviewing, both for a residency placement, but also for a hospital staff position or to win acceptance for a fellowship, your aim is to make a positive impression and to stand out in a good way from the other candidates. Here are my recommendations for upping your odds at having a great interview.

Information Gathering

If possible, find out the full names of the people who will be interviewing you and do an internet search to gather background information about them. Try to learn their current positions in the organization, the relationship of their positions to the one you are applying for, the length of time they've spent at the organization, the various positions they may have held already within the organization, and other organizations they may have worked with. The more you know about them, the more you can use that to your advantage during your interview by asking certain questions or framing your responses in a way they'd likely find agreeable. If possible try to communicate with other employees before the interview to find out about the personalities of your interviewers and also the general culture of the place. The more knowledge you have going into the interview, the more prepared, competent, and agreeable you can show yourself to be.

Professional Dress

A frequent complaint that medical employers have is the attire that prospective medical staff, including consulting positions, wear to the interview. Apparently, it isn't uncommon for interviewees to dress too casually, wearing sweatshirts, jeans, or even scrubs.

Be sure to dress professionally for your interview. It's better to be too professional in your dress and get it wrong than too casual. Opt for business professional attire to show respect for your interviewers and the organization you are aiming to join.

Reconsider Caffeine

Because you'll likely already be amped up, it can be a good idea not to drink coffee or ingest any kind of caffeine before the interview. Some candidates appear too zippy, overly talkative, or sweaty if they have coffee before an interview. You want to appear calm, focused, smart, and professional—everything that a supercharge from caffeine can take away from you!

Timeliness

Of course, arriving late to your interview is a bad idea, but arriving too early isn't good either. Sometimes interview candidates arrive 20 to 60 minutes early for their interviews, and staff tend to not like it. They get uncomfortable thinking there must be some kind of miscommunication about the start time of the interview.

If you arrive super early to your interview, don't go inside the building. Find somewhere to wait inconspicuously and only five or ten minutes beforehand, enter the building.

General Courtesy

Expect everyone at the organization to be watching you and taking note of your behavior and level of professionalism. The front desk person, the receptionist—anyone who works for the organization is likely going to be asked by the interviewers to give their impression of you. Be courteous to everyone.

Be a Starter

When you see the interviewers coming towards you, be sure to stand immediately and extend your arm to shake hands. Don't sit there—knowing who they are but waiting for them to initiate things. You'll come off as passive. Instead, you want to come off as enthusiastic and confident (but not bossy). The interviewer will notice your positive, can-do attitude.

Ice Breaker

If possible, check out the surroundings to see if there are photos or something else indicating the interviewers' interests. You might realize they like water skiing, ceramics, or that they have young children. The point is to find something from their life that you can ask a question about to break the ice and establish a rapport. Also, later on when you write your follow-up "thank-you" note, you can mention this topic of interest again. It'll make your note more personal and less generic.

Targeted Responses

Because most interviews involve some variation of "Tell me about yourself," be sure to tailor your response to that question—and to all questions—to also explain why you are a great fit for the position you are interviewing for. For instance, rather than answering, "I'm a huge LA Lakers fan, and I enjoy ice skating," say something along the lines of, "I love traveling internationally, particularly when I can do international medical work. Just last month, I was doing medical work in a remote village of Mexico, helping indigenous people who can't afford medical care. It was very rewarding." Try to redirect questions to your relevant talents and abilities as smoothly as possible.

Down-to-Earth and Real

The most successful interviewees talk in a real, down-to-earth way. They draw from stories from their own lives and specific examples. The least successful interviewees use a lot of jargon, a lot of buzzwords, speaking in generalities but without much substance. Something else to avoid is repeatedly using filler-type words, "Um," "Yeah," "So," "You know," and such. Though using these kinds of filler words might just be a sign of nervousness, it can make you look unprofessional and unpolished.

It is more effective to credit your department and team than to attribute yourself as the achiever in obviously team achievements. Interviewees, who acknowledge their part in a group, and how together that group was able to reach success, do far better than interviewees who are constantly praising themselves and using "I" and "me" a lot. No matter your medical specialty, you won't be working alone. You'll have supporting staff and fellow doctors that you'll be working with, so be sure to show that you recognize the team effort when you cite achievements from your past.

Always Professional

When you are at the location of the job interview, maintain your most professional comportment. Never back down from being professional even if you are in a different part of the building or campus, in a restroom, walking a hallway, or in a courtyard. It's been said that an interviewing physician was speaking on the phone in the outdoor area of the hospital, critiquing the hospital's layout. Little did they know that the receptionist was also outside taking a five-minute break in the fresh air. That person wasn't offered a position.

A Thank You

After the interview, be sure to send a follow-up message—either by email or mail—thanking the interviewers as well as including another personal comment regarding a topic of interest that came up in the interview. If you smoothly finesse this thank you + comment, it can work really well in your favor.

While this chapter addresses the residency interview, the next chapter turns to residency itself. It's a burdensome few years. Incredibly difficult. Very grueling. But it's what you've been preparing for and you know you can make it. The next chapter delivers a few recommendations on how to make your residency years a bit more manageable.

As a bonus with this book, you will receive physician interview questions and answers (and much more) by signing up to www.myfellowship.com for free and contacting Dr. Mohy Taha through the platform.

Chapter 18

Residency Survival Kit

A s you've likely heard, residency is going to be a grueling period. For the few who say it isn't, they are posturing. Don't believe them. On all levels—mental, physical, and emotional—residency is going to exhaust you. Yes, there will be some brief highlights, but you can't predict when those will happen. And, as I've said, the rewards they offer will be brief. What makes the exhaustion and toil of residency worth it is the depth of skills and experience you will gain. It is mind-blowing. However, to survive it and come out the other side to practice all that you learn for decades to come—it's going to be tough. Here are my recommendations for making the best of that difficult time.

Cultivate Positivity

There is so little you can control during this tough period—your schedule, your hours, your cases, your supervisors and staff, so much is out of your hands. But the one thing you have ownership over is the attitude and perspective you bring with you. It is up to you to choose to take it in stride and find the positives or to be like so many others and concentrate on the negatives. This isn't something that happens once, choosing a positive mindset is something you have to actively cultivate, again and again, in an attempt to make it your go-to take on your days. But you can do it. Harness the one thing you can control—and decide to see the positives in this difficult time. It'll make it more bearable, which can make all the difference in terms of surviving.

Remember Your Own Health

Just like you might be helping your patients to see, your own health isn't something you take care of on the go. Just like your patients, your health is the result of many small daily-life decisions you make. For example, exercise, healthy eating, adequate sleeping—making regular time in your hectic residency for these, from day one, could save you from mental and physical burnout. Make it a priority to do all you can to support yourself mentally and physically so that you have the reserves to best endure residency.

Depression, anxiety, and stress are not uncommon for residents/registrars to land in due to the incredible demands of residency. Just as you would advise a patient, don't accept a consistently dangerous mental state as not a big deal. Don't brush it off. Ask for help if you need it. Surviving residency, the rest of your career, or even your life could depend on it.

Invest in Your Relationships

Realistically, you won't be able to spend the same amount of time with your friends and family as before, but even still—don't let those relationships crumble. It's important to check in with your supporting relationships as much as you can during your residency. Don't make promises you can't keep—like spending the weekend with them if you know it's not going to happen. Be realistic in what you can offer, but don't let them slide. They will help you reset and remember the big picture. They will listen to you and make you feel supported amidst your exhaustion. They provide an important outlet for you during a trying time. Me and Madleina were very lucky to have Christian and Annelis Ludwig (my parents in law) who supported us countless hours looking after our children.

I should mention too that your fellow residents are the people you are going to be spending the most time with during your residency years. You all will be together a lot, and you all are the only ones who totally get what you are each enduring. Sometimes you will not get along. Sometimes you'll feel like soul mates. Do all you can to embrace your fellow residents. Getting irritated at them, constantly fighting with them—it only makes your already difficult job worse. Just like you can choose a positive attitude, you can choose to accept your fellow residents—and maybe even like them too!

Keep It Real

If someone asks you something—and you don't know—keep it real with them and say, "I don't know." You are not expected to know everything. As a matter of fact, you are expected to be honest. When you don't know, you can then suggest, "I can try to find out if you point me in the right direction." Whether it's a nurse, a patient, a fellow resident, or your supervisor—you will likely get asked questions that you regularly just don't know the answer to. And that's okay. It shows greater depth, honesty, and professionalism on your part to admit what you don't know and try to make an effort to find out than to pretend you know. So do the right thing and be real with yourself and with others.

Better and Better

While all of residency is tough, it gets increasingly less tough (but still tough) over time. What I mean is that the beginning is the worst. That's when it's most overwhelming. But after a few months, you will realize that it isn't as all-out awful as it was at the start. This slight easing up of the difficulty happens over the course of your residency.

You see, at the start it is all brand new—even figuring out the configuration of the hospital is new. People's names. What they do and don't do; know and don't know. Over time, you figure out the things that at the start add up to make it all so new and overwhelming. You'll accumulate some wins in diagnosing and treating common illnesses. While you will never get enough sleep, you'll get a bit used to functioning on less sleep. As long as you do your very best to take care of your health during your residency, with each passing day it gets a bit better—and you'll look back and realize how far along you've come as a physician. You'll survive, and you'll be proud.

While I doubt my recommendations have struck awe in you, that's fine. It's expected. You've endured so much already to make it to residency—remember that. Remember that you are a fighter and that you are prepared. This is what you've been training for, so do it. Do your very best. You are preparing yourself for a lifetime of important work.

And once you've completed residency, I hope you don't see that as an end to your training. Not at all! To give yourself the much-needed practice in your subspecialty, in order to become a true expert, I advocate doing an international fellowship. Remember the "fellowship triangle"? This triangle highlights the three big benefits of doing a fellowship–training, mentorship, and traveling. Give yourself access to the three legs of this triangle—do an international fellowship! The next chapter outlines how to apply to one.

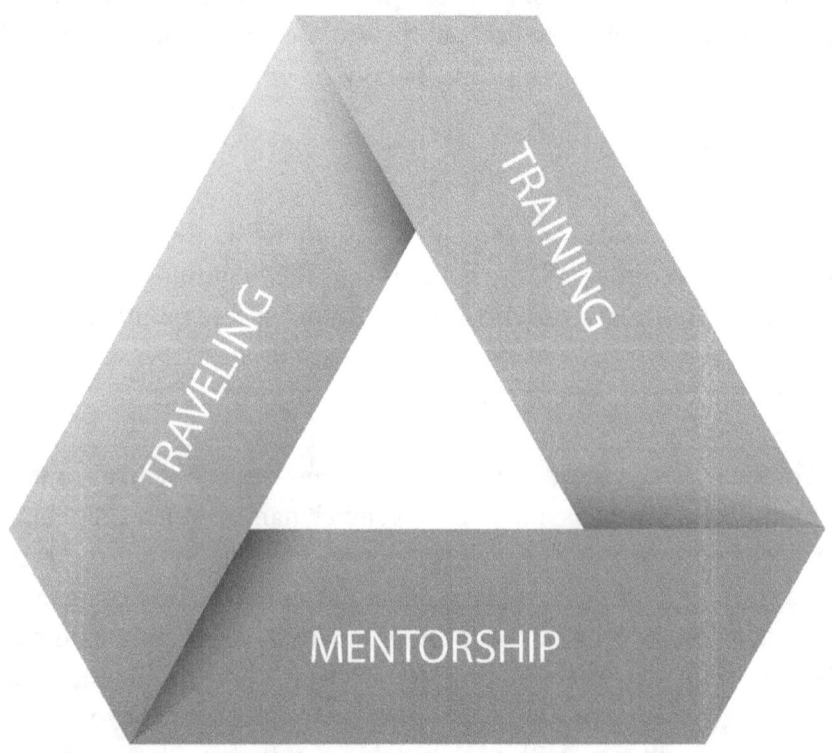

Fellow

Medical Career Success Path

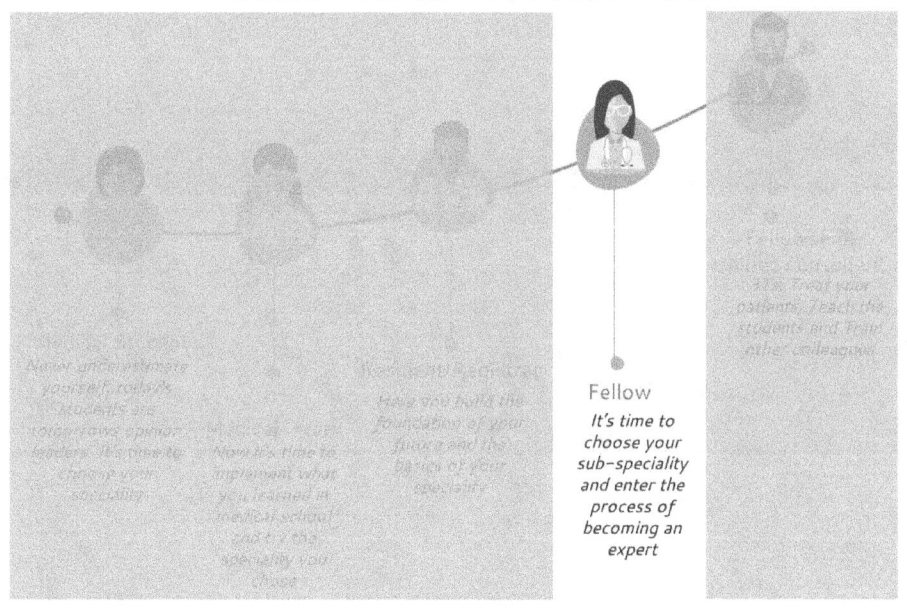

Fellow

It's time to choose your sub-speciality and enter the process of becoming an expert

Chapter 19

Tips on Applying for Fellowships

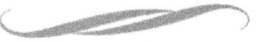

Optimizing Your Chances

If you consider the trajectory of the medical career success path, you'll notice that I applied to do fellowships in Australia starting immediately after I completed my time as a resident/registrar. Even though it might have been more convenient for me and my family financially if I spent the first few years, after residency, moonlighting at various hospitals and clinics to work off some debt and ease our financial strain, I knew that I'd have a better chance at landing fellowships if I applied while I was still in training. If you wait too long to apply for a fellowship after your training has finished, fellowship providers won't see you as relevant or the most desirable. So to stay relevant and increase your chances at landing fellowships, even if it isn't financially convenient, it's best to apply while you are still in residency and to apply with the aim of starting the fellowship soon after your residency ends. Another good idea too is to spend a year as chief resident or junior consultant. This will boost your status when applying to fellowships.

Where to Apply

As I've recommended multiple times, start your fellowship search using the database at www.myfellowship.com.

Using the filters provided on this platform will help you locate fellowships that could be very relevant to your needs. From there, once you've narrowed it down, you can read the reviews of current and past fellows (mentors) and even contact them to ask them specific questions—all of which should help you determine if the fellowship seems a good fit for you. As well, you should go to the fellowship's website and read all you can there. In your own residency program, you can talk to co-residents and mentors, as well, to find out about fellowships they might have done or that they know about. Perhaps they can give you further information on promising fellowships you found on MY-FELLOWSHIP as well. If your institution offers a relevant fellowship, apply to it as well. Especially if you've made good connections with your supervisors and performed well during your residency, you'll have a great chance of landing a fellowship at your own institution, though, of course, if you can get an international fellowship—I'd recommend taking that one first!

While the daily life issues shouldn't determine which fellowship you accept, you still need to take them into account. For instance, if you have a family and they are coming with you during your fellowship, they must be reasonably happy to spend the year or so in that new place. You have to take into account the kind of schools your kids could go to, perhaps even the language, culture, and values of the new place. Younger kids can adjust more easily to new and amazing adventures while older kids may be more interested in staying with their group of friends in their home country. If your spouse has a thriving career in your home country, they might not be interested in taking a leave. It isn't uncommon for a temporary family separation to happen to make a fellowship happen. This happened with my family, who only spent six months, of the 1.5 years I was in Australia, with me. You need to figure out beforehand what you and your family can handle because if the circumstances end up too stressful, then it will take a toll on your abilities to train in the fellowship. Your fellowship lasts only a year or a few years, but it will greatly affect the rest of your career as a consulting physician.

Be sure to check over all the prerequisites before making the effort to apply to a fellowship. If there's a requirement that you simply don't meet, say even a visa requirement, then you don't want to waste your time applying.

The Application Process

If you'll recall from my fellowship application, I began applying two years before I intended to start. I urge you to get started early with these. Notice deadlines and the timing for specialty matches. When you decide on your specialty, make sure to do the electives, cultivate relationships with mentors in that specialty, and even do research in it way before applying to the fellowship. That way when you do apply, you show yourself as a strong candidate. If your mentors agree to be your references, as Professor Gerber was for me, it only increases your chances of gaining placement.

You don't have to wait for the deadline to submit your application. In fact, you shouldn't. Institutions begin looking at applications as they come in, so it could be better to be among the first, weeks before the deadline, than to wait on the day of the deadline when they receive several hundred.

Similar to my recommendations for the residency interview, be truthful on your application. Don't exaggerate your knowledge, skills, or your role in research. Acknowledge when it wasn't just you, but a whole team effort—a team that you were a member of—that achieved something. If you inflate yourself in a key area, it will be evident during the interview (assuming you make it there) when you are speaking with an expert in the area.

Your application should also include aspects of yourself beyond medicine—your areas of interest, special life experiences, hobbies, and such. You want to present yourself as a whole person with a larger story—rather than an anonymous myopically-focused medicine machine. Of course, you should frame all these additional facets of yourself to show how they advance your abilities and interests in medicine. It's a careful balance. And you need to keep all this writing short too. If you aren't a great writer, be ready to hire an outside editor to help you with the writing.

As already stated, I had a big name in my orthopedics and traumatology specialty, Professor Christian Gerber, serve as my reference. The reason this worked is that he and I knew each other well and worked closely. It's actually better to have your reference be someone who knows you well and has worked closely with you than simply be a big name in your specialty. If you are like me and you have someone who is both—then great. But, if you vaguely know a prominent specialist but a much less prominent one knows you really well and supports you, then the latter is who you should go with. It's much more impressive to fellowship providers to hear from a reference who can cite specific examples of the work you've done and who knows you and speaks warmly and highly of you—than to read what a big name specialist has to say—which often isn't much.

The Interview

Don't be annoying to the fellowship provider once you've submitted your application. For instance, it is fine to call one time to confirm that the application you submitted is complete and has been reviewed. But don't ask the administrator about your chances for landing an interview because that person likely won't know—and they might even be moved to mark your file as someone who is questionable.

If you do make it to the interview round, be sure to respond to that contact. Accept a given interview date and time, or if you've already decided to discontinue applying to the fellowship, state that. If something comes up and you must change your interview date and time, give as much advanced notice as possible. Actually, do all you can not to make any changes because it could be looked at as selfish and unprofessional, especially if it is last minute. Something to realize is that, even if you don't intend on pursuing the fellowship, you should remain helpful and courteous at all times. Don't be rude or simply disappear on the program. It's a small world and down the line you may have another important interaction with this program or program director (they might move to another institution that you are interested in), so you want to stand out as a courteous and professional person. Not as thoughtless and rude.

Similar to my recommendations for the residency interview, plan early how you'll travel to your fellowship interview. Arrive five to ten minutes early, but not way earlier than that. Dress professionally in conservative business attire. It's better to be overdressed than underdressed. Be considerate to everyone you interact with in the institution—from the front-desk person to the window washer. Behave as if you assume everyone is watching and evaluating you. So even in the restroom or outside the building, be careful what you say on your cellphone. You want to make a good impression on all the staff. If you stand out as negative in any way, it could be your downfall—even if you think your interview with the higher-ups goes fine.

When it is time for the interview, be sure to stand, offer your hand in a firm handshake, and make eye contact with the interviewers when they approach. Don't stay seated and force them to initiate it all. You'll come off as passive and unenthusiastic—the opposite of how you want to appear (and how you should be feeling at the chance to do a fellowship). When you take your seat with the interviewer, continue looking them in the eye and showing you are interested and enthusiastic. Don't look at your feet, look out the window, or look just past the interviewer. Also, show you are prepared and eager.

As far as preparation goes—before arriving, consider a few interesting patient cases you have come across in your years in residency that you think are relevant to your fellowship. Prepare yourself to talk about these cases in detail. Nothing is worse and more awkward than a fellowship interviewee who has spent four-plus years in residency and cannot come up with a single relevant patient case. If you have done research, prepare yourself to talk about that research. Make sure to be able to discuss its background and details. Don't think you can just remember it all on the fly. You'll be talking with an expert in your interview, and they will be fully aware of any inconsistencies on your part. Another part of preparation is the questions you'll be asking. Be careful if your questions concentrate on the amount of work the fellowship entails. You don't want to come off as afraid to work hard. Instead ask questions that show you've thought deeply about the nature of the work, the nuances of it. This will require you to know something about the work involved in the fellowship, but I would think if you've been following my advice throughout this whole book and combing MY-FELLOWSHIP about this fellowship, reading reviews from current and previous fellows and contacting them with follow-up questions—that you will enter the interview with a solid picture of the nature of the fellowship work and will have a lot of applicable questions already prepared.

After the interview, when you send a thank-you note to the interviewers, be sure it is personal. Be sure to spell their names correctly and make a comment that shows you aren't writing a "form" email.

About Acceptance

Because some specialties are very competitive to land fellowships in, you might want to consider applying to a fellowship outside of your specialty. It is possible too for a fellowship to accept an applicant whose specialty doesn't match their own. Know this is a possibility in case you find yourself in a competitive specialty with limited options.

As tempting as it can be to do otherwise, rank your fellowship based on the ones you most want, rather than the ones you predict you'll most likely get accepted into. Also, many applicants don't realize this, but it's no longer necessary to call the program director of your top choice fellowship to let them know it's your top choice. This is no longer normal practice. However, if you can't help yourself and you truly will take the fellowship if it's offered to you, it won't necessarily hurt you to make the call or even to have your resident supervisor call for you. However, if in the end, this fellowship is offered to you but you don't take it, you will be greatly discredited. Both your own resident supervisor and the program director will likely hold it against you and consider you unprofessional and an opportunist. Remember, this could likely hurt you later on because the world of medicine, particularly in your specialty, isn't a big one.

If you'll recall, in chapter 16 I explained how I went to Australia to interview for several fellowships. The next chapter explains how even in the midst of planning for the yearlong fellowships in Australia, I also applied for and completed a shorter fellowship, in Brazil. We'll take a look at that and then return to the Australian fellowships in chapter 21.

All revenue generated from this book will be donated to the community platform: www.myfellowship.com

Chapter 20
The Brazilian Samba: From Rio to Manaus

H ere's another important reason to do an international fellowship: for those of us training in highly developed countries, like Switzerland, we often don't encounter the challenges that doctors training in developing countries must be adept at handling. As a result, our repertoire is limited, and we miss out on some important training experiences. For instance, medical systems in developing countries often must contend with a lack of equipment (plates, screws, instruments), overcrowded hospitals, and unhygienic conditions. Even the types of diseases, injuries, and such can greatly differ in developed versus developing countries.

The Swiss medical system is a very expensive system, and it functions well. However, I figured it would be beneficial to see how to practice medicine on around one-tenth of the budget and still deliver an acceptable medical service. For this reason, even as I was planning out the year-long fellowship in Australia, I decided I'd like to experience trauma surgery in a developing country. That's why I decided to go to Brazil to do another fellowship. And if we think to the international fellowship triangle, the other two sides of it—mentors and traveling— also played a part!

Let me tell you how mentorship played a role in my pursuing this fellowship opportunity. During the AO Foundation courses in Davos, I met Professor Mauricio Kfuri, who hailed from Ribeirão Preto, Brazil. Professor Kfuri became a mentor of mine, and I was able to spend six weeks in a trauma fellowship provided by the AO Foundation with him in Ribeirão Preto, Brazil.

Just to clarify the timing, before I spent a year in Australia doing two fellowships (2016), when I was still making plans for that year-long Australian fellowship experience and finishing my final year of residency (2015), that's when I did this six-week fellowship in Brazil.

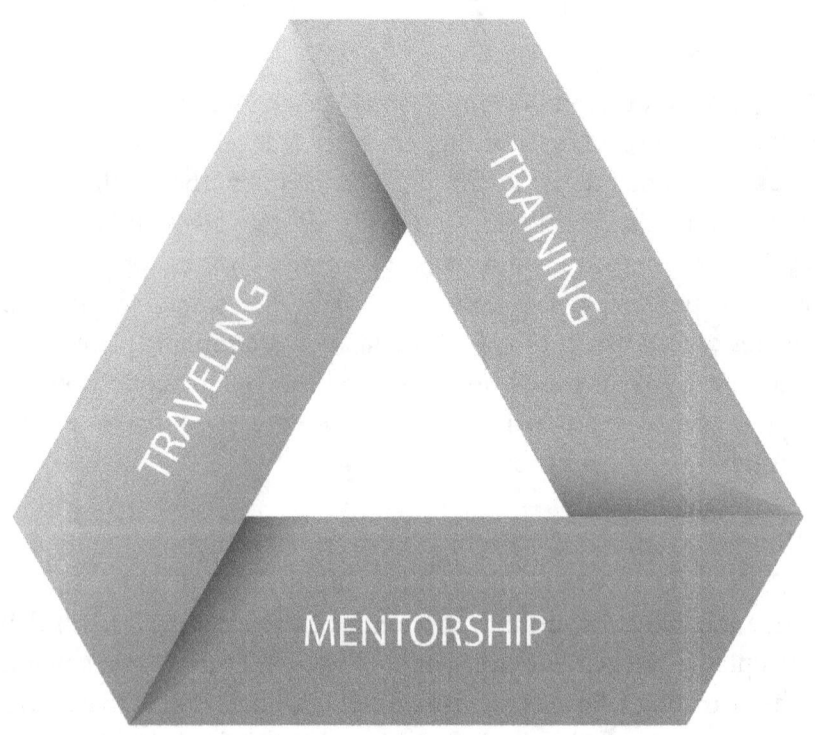

Fellowship Triangle: Training Side

On the medical level, my time in fellowship in Brazil was incredibly fruitful. I saw very interesting cases and got immersed in the Brazilian medical system. I was assigned to Dr. Tavares, a consultant in Professor Kfuri's team, and I joined different operations with him in different hospitals. Also, the whole team made me feel at home, Professor Fabricio Fogagnolo, the consultants, as well as the residents. I saw a lot of types of implants that we no longer use in Europe, implants that have been replaced by more expensive, high-tech models, but these other implants are still being used in Brazil. The dynamic hip screw (DHS) is one of these examples. In Europe it is rarely used now due to the availably of intra-medullary nails. Though DHS isn't as fancy or as minimally invasive, it still works well. Some of the interesting cases included the "blade plate" for proximal femur fracture mal-union or non-union accompanied by an osteotomy. Also, the use of Ilizarov external fixator (Ilizarov frame) was interesting. Moreover, in the emergency department, I was exposed to multiple polytrauma (multiple traumata) patients.

Fellowship Triangle: Mentorship Side

Through Professor Kfuri, I got invited to the University Hospital of Manaus to visit Dr. Chang, the head of the traumatology and orthopedics department there. Through my fellowship I learned a lot from Professor Kfuri, Dr. Tavares, Professor Fogagnolo, and Dr. Chang, both professionally and personally, which expanded my personal network to include mentors in South America.

Fellowship Triangle: Travel Side

Traveling in Brazil was sensational. I went to Rio de Janeiro and São Paulo. I visited Manaus, and from there got to tour the Amazon River and rainforest. I even traveled to see Iguazú Falls, which makes up the largest system of waterfalls in the world.

While this Brazilian fellowship immersed me in the three benefits of the "fellowship triangle," training, mentorship, and traveling, this was only a taster! The next chapter describes my preparation for the Australian yearlong fellowship as well as a description of that awesome experience. And remember, I'm describing all this to excite you to enter the world of discovery that international opportunities offer us at pretty much every stage on our medical career paths!

Chapter 21

Overcoming Challenges for a Worthwhile Fellowship

L et's return to the Australian fellowship. As already explained, I was super excited to get the fellowship offer. However, something I learned was that getting these offers didn't mean an end to the difficult and intense planning. In a lot of ways, that's when the planning became most challenging! That's the subject of this chapter—the additional challenges you have to overcome to make your fellowship offer materialize. For me, these challenges were in terms of paperwork, financials, organizing daily-life issues, and timing.

Paperwork Hurdles

Being accepted into the fellowship doesn't mean you can go. There remains heaps and heaps and heaps of paperwork to get through: to understand the medical system in a foreign country, to register to get permission to practice there, to get a visa there (and get visas for your family if they'll be coming with you), and if the language of your documents and that of the country you want to do fellowship in differ, there's the translation and notarizing of all of the documents.

Australia had extensive and strict regulations. For example, they needed official translations of original certificates, like my medical school diploma. As mine was from Egypt and in Arabic, a certified translator translated it into English and put stamps on it. Then a notary had to notarize it too. Then we sent it to Australia to be checked. A month or six weeks later, when the Australian officials checked it, they ended up turning it down because the official translator wrote, "This is a translation from the original" but didn't write, "This is a correct translation from the original." I would have thought that the fact it was an official translation, anyone could assume it to be correctly translated, but because this word wasn't written on it, it didn't count. So, it had to be done again. This cost a lot of money, time, and effort.

Because of requirements like this, having a current fellow who can give you tips for navigating the process really helps.

It took me seven months to do all the paperwork. It was such a tricky process that I actually wrote a guide on it, A Roadmap to Australian Fellowships, available on Amazon.com for anyone interested. https://www.amazon.com/Roadmap-Australian-Fellowships-Mohy-Taha-ebook/dp/B07MPR58QD. Here are the issues that guide covers:

- The visa and accreditation requirements
- The "documents parcel": all about original and certified documents
- Everything to do in the final month before leaving for Australia
- Everything to have prepared to enter Australia
- What to do after you've entered to set yourself up
- Expected costs for registration/paperwork
- Options for your leisure time to enjoy Australia

I know I'm repeating myself, but this is such an important point that I'm making it again: this process is so incredibly involved that you must do the legwork beforehand to make sure that the fellowship(s) you ultimately do are worth the effort, time, energy, and expense required to do them. And key to that is connecting with current and past fellows. Also, current and past fellows can also give you advice and support in handling the huge paperwork (and social) hurdles. For example, a current or past fellow can help you with these questions:

- Australia requires a "certificate of good practice," something that doesn't exist in Switzerland. What advice do you have on handling this?
- Where to look to rent an apartment?
- Where to live in terms of schools for children?
- Where's a good place to get a used car?
- As not every hospital has good reception for all cellular signals, for instance, Vodafone might work well but Telstra not so much, any advice for this issue?

Reaching out to current and previous fellows provides you some significant shortcuts.

Financial Hurdles

Depending on where you want to do your fellowship, you might be dealing with a country that is very expensive. That was certainly the case with Australia. If you find yourself in this situation, you really must figure out the finances beforehand or else you'll be left in financial crisis during the fellowship and/or in debt afterward.

Something that I find incredibly backward is how grants for research are more readily available than financial support to do fellowships. To me this is odd because fellowships teach doctors the skills that they'll be applying immediately and for years to come, yet it is very difficult to find grants and aid to fund fellowships. On the other hand, many foundations and organizations give grants for research even though the findings of that research might never amount to anything or there might be decades of delay before the findings are implemented to even a small degree.

I find it frustrating that there's such little financial support available to fellowships especially in comparison to all the money out there to fund research. What you learn from a fellowship has a direct influence on the patient care from the day you finish your fellowship. You go back home and apply the skills you learned. To me, the importance of financially supporting fellowships has been underestimated.

Because of the scarcity of funding options, sometimes a fellow has to live on savings during their time in fellowship, or they go into debt to finance the year of fellowship learning. This financial issue is one that MY-FELLOWSHIP is seeking to solve. MY-FELLOWSHIP seeks sponsors to provide financial support for aspiring fellows. One problem I've encountered is that when I've asked companies if they can donate money to support fellows, they say it isn't possible because of compliance regulations. They cannot give money to any doctor directly. That's why we formed the organization behind MY-FELLOWSHIP. Companies can contribute to our organization, and in turn the organization can use this money to help any doctor who is accepted for a fellowship and is looking for financial support. This is yet another reason I urge medical students, aspiring fellows, etc., to visit MY-FELLOWSHIP. It's another resource we offer to help aspiring fellows overcome the obstacles to make a fellowship happen.

Daily Life Issues

There are many daily life issues to sort out when leaving to pursue a fellowship for a year. If you own a house, condo, car, or office, you must determine what will happen with those while you are away. For my wife and me, we had a home in Switzerland, and we had a mortgage we'd have to pay, so it would help us to rent it out while we were away. Plus, as a pediatrician, she had her own private office space and had to find someone to see her patients while she was away. Moreover, we had to find an Australian school for our children.

Timing

It's also not always easy to time your fellowship. For instance, for my fellowship, I was applying to start in July 2016, but then they informed me that they had a position in January free. I agreed to take it because I worried I'd risk losing the fellowship otherwise. Starting six months earlier than originally planned raised other timing issues. For instance, with a January start, my wife and children wouldn't be able to join me and stay for a full year. Instead, they could only join me in July (thus, stay with me in Australia for a half-year).

A second timing issue was an important Swiss training exam in June. I realized I'd have to return to Switzerland to take it. We arranged that I would return in June to take the exam and see my family. Then I would go back to Australia to continue the fellowship. Two weeks later, my family would join me for the first time in Australia.

In November of that year, I returned to Switzerland again to take oral exams (and my family stayed in Australia). Then I flew back to Australia to complete the final two months of the Sydney part of the fellowship. In January we all returned to Switzerland, but then I went back again to Australia, going to Brisbane to do five months of fellowship there. My family didn't return with me because it was too hard to swing financially. Even during these five months, I returned to Switzerland to see my family once.

It was a lot of mileage coming and going during that fellowship. And each time I was back in Switzerland I was doing interviews for my physician consultant job I'd start once the fellowship ended. It wasn't easy organizing these interviews from the other side of the world, but with good organization and communication—plus serious drive—it was possible.

Domestic vs. Foreign Fellowship

It isn't uncommon for doctors to do fellowships at a different and new location within their own countries, which are called "domestic" fellowships. Of course, this saves a lot of the headaches I've described that go along with foreign fellowships. While it is certainly a viable option, depending on your goals and circumstances, it might not make sense for you to do a domestic fellowship.

For me, doing a fellowship in Switzerland didn't make sense. I had already worked in three different hospitals with the top Swiss experts in my subspecialty of the shoulder and elbow. Thus, there weren't any new hospitals or new mentors for me. And if you think of the three parts of the fellowship triangle—training, mentors, and traveling—already I'd met the mentors and done the training (and traveling too) in Switzerland. However, all three parts of that triangle were open for me when it came to the rest of the world, particularly training in that I would get to see more patients and do more shoulder and elbow surgeries. Because I'm someone who loves traveling and is constantly building relationships, international fellowships were ideal for me.

It was ideal for my family too. My wife and I really wanted our children to have the experience of going to school in another language. In the case of Australia, an English-speaking school with English-speaking teachers and friends. When my children arrived in Australia, they didn't speak any English. After three months, they were already speaking fluent Aussie. In the end, the Australian fellowship was a win-win for me professionally and for my family.

My Australian Fellowship

Though I didn't have MY-FELLOWSHIP to help me, I put in enough effort beforehand so that the fellowships I did in Australia ended up being interesting and rewarding experiences. I commenced the fellowship in January 2016, and throughout the year worked under the expert guidance of the esteemed Dr. Benjamin Cass, Dr. Allan Young, and Dr. Jeffery Hughes, as well as in close contact with Professor David Sonnabend, who was in semi-retirement. Assisting more than 500 operations in three different private hospitals with three different consultants exposed me to a great variety of techniques and implants, and helped develop my problem-solving skills during the different operations. Carrying out more than 70 operations by myself in three public hospitals also improved my surgical skills in open, arthroscopic shoulder and elbow surgeries.

Through cooperation with the biomechanics and biomedical devices departments of the University of Sydney, I was also able to complete two research projects. Furthermore, I gave two oral presentations, one at the Royal North Shore Shoulder Symposium and the other at the Shoulder and Elbow Society of Australia Conference in Darwin.

On the social level you also meet fellows and consultants from around the globe and even sometimes from your own country. For instance my co-fellow was Dr. Gregory Cunningham from Geneva, who I met for the first time during my fellowship and we developed a great friendship. I also got introduced to PD Dr. Alexandre Laedermann who also works in Geneva as a shoulder and elbow consultant and the founder of www.beemed.com, which is the first participative medical education platform. MY-FELLOWSHIP and Beemed believe in the mission of each other and support it.

In summary, this fellowship experience was a milestone in my career and gave me the training in shoulder and elbow surgery I'd hoped for. The next year after the fellowship, when I started my career in Switzerland as a consulting physician with a subspecialty in shoulder and elbow surgery, I was confident about the expertise I was offering my patients.

Because a foreign fellowship requires such an investment of time, effort, and money to organize in the months (or two years, as in my case) before it starts, you must be sure, before actually starting it, that the fellowship you are interested in is right for you. Do all you can to make a good choice for which fellowship(s) you're going to apply to because it has lots of consequences on your career and your financial situation.

Make sure it's worth the whole process of pre-planning and worth the actual year you'll spend doing it. MY-FELLOWSHIP, www.myfellowship.com, offers resources to help you make the most informed decision about a fellowship, so use those resources. In addition to fellowships, MY-FELLOWSHIP also offers in-depth information about observerships. Let's take a look at observerships.

Observerships

MY-FELLOWSHIP not only offers important insights into

finding the right fellowship(s) for your needs, but it also offers crucial information about observerships. It is an open-source encyclopedia so everyone is welcomed to share their observership and feedback about it. An observership is essentially a very short fellowship. It can last a few days to a month. You do not do an observership to learn a lot of skills. You do an observership to learn about something specific, new products being put to use, new techniques, or one new procedure. As with the longer fellowship (which can last several months to a year), you can do domestic or international observerships that allow you to seize all three sides of the "fellowship triangle": training, mentors, and traveling. Observerships give you the opportunity to travel around the world to expand your learning under the mentorship of experts.

If you'll recall from my own medical journey, I've done a number of observerships. For instance, as noted in chapter 5, when I was in my third year of medical school in Cairo, I participated in a four-week medical exchange, thus an observership, in Berlin, Germany at Charité–Universitätsmedizin (Charity University Hospital). During the observership, I connected with Dr. Stahel, who later gave approval for me to spend a year at his lab doing research (while I was also learning the German language). Notice from this example, it was a short international exchange that offered me new learning and mentorship and exposed me to Germany (and Europe) for the first time. I loved it, and it set me up to do more observerships and fellowships during medical school, residency, and even after I became a consulting physician.

Since becoming a consulting physician, I've done many fruitful observerships, including among them are the following:

- January 2017—Clinique La Colline, Geneva, Switzerland with PD Dr. Alexandre Lädermann
- March 2018—Clinique Generale, Anncey, France with Dr. Laurent Lafosse
- October 2018—Tampa General Hospital, Tampa, Florida, USA with Dr. Mark Frankle
- March 2019—Massachusetts General Hospital, Harvard, Boston,

Massachusetts, USA with Professor J. Warner and Dr. Luke Oh

- March 2019—Mayo Clinic, Rochester, New York, USA with Dr. M. Morrey and Prof. B. Elhassan
- March 2019—St. Joseph Hospital, Toronto, Ontario, Canada with Prof. G. Athwal

As you can see, I've made the effort to expand my abilities and learning through these observerships as well as expanding my network and all the while experiencing new cities, countries, and cultures. With observerships, you can do this too. You'll find in your medical career that at conferences, you meet a lot of experts who have developed specific techniques that are very pertinent to you and your work. Through an observership, you can visit an expert to expand your own expertise in a specific technique. Perhaps your stay with them is for a couple of days, to a couple of weeks.

When you participate in observerships, you expand your network, which not only serves you but serves your trainees as well. Through your new relationships with these experts you give your trainees access to a new hospital or clinic where they too can go and visit, spend some time in an observership, or even do a full-time fellowship.

MY-FELLOWSHIP is ripe with opportunities and the nuanced information behind those opportunities to help you and your colleagues, trainees, and residents locate the most pertinent, beneficial, and interesting opportunities—whether fellowships or observerships—that will end up forging important across-the-world relationships, such that many doctors and patient communities will, in turn, benefit. I can't encourage you enough to make use of the MY-FELLOWSHIP platform. If you would like to know more about how MY-FELLOWSHIP can help your medical career or what you can do to contribute, please visit us at www.myfellowship.com.

In the next chapter I share the three important areas of concentration where, as a consulting physician, you will spend the length of your career focusing on. I call these three areas, the "three Ts."

Fellowship Trained Consultant

Medical Career Success Path

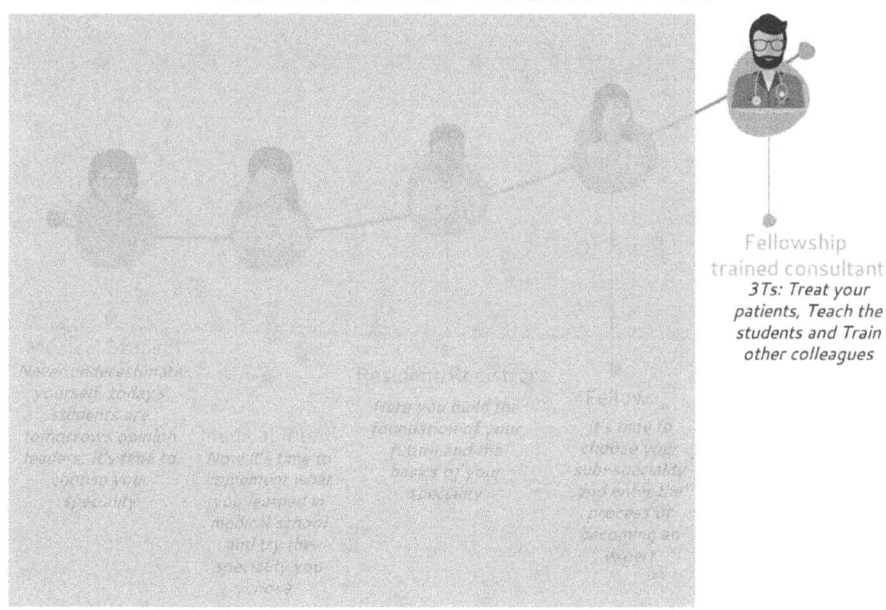

Fellowship
trained consultant
*3Ts: Treat your
patients, Teach the
students and Train
other colleagues*

Never underestimate
yourself, today's
students are
tomorrows opinion
leaders. It's time to
choose your
speciality

Medical school
Now it's time to
implement what
you learned in
medical school
and try the
speciality you
loved

Residency is going
help you build the
foundations of your
future and the
basics of your
speciality

Fellow
It's time to
choose your
sub-speciality
and enjoy the
process of
becoming an
expert

Chapter 22
The Three Ts

After completing residency and your fellowship(s), during which time you get the training you need to become an expert in your chosen subspecialty, you become a consulting physician, i.e., a consultant. It's not the end when you finish your training and start working as a consultant. It's only the beginning of the real work, where you will use all of the training and experience you've collected through your education, training, and fellowship(s) to start a new phase as an expert.

As a consultant, there are three major areas–the "three Ts"–that I, along with many other consultants, have identified as the focus of the consulting physician's career. The first T is treating your patients. Naturally, treating your patients is a main part of your job. The second T is teaching up-and-coming medical students. Just as a variety of mentors supported you, and likely will continue to support you, you will provide mentorship, both formal and informal, for doctors in training. You will empower the new generation and teach them. The third T is comprised of training your colleagues, which is part of the job, as well, training new residents/registrars and fellows. You will provide training and guidance to all of the people who are assisting you, similar to how your mentors did for you when you were in residency, fellowship(s), and observership(s).

As I see it, a consultant functions in these three parts, i.e., the "three Ts":

1. Treat your patient.
2. Teach students.
3. Train your colleagues.

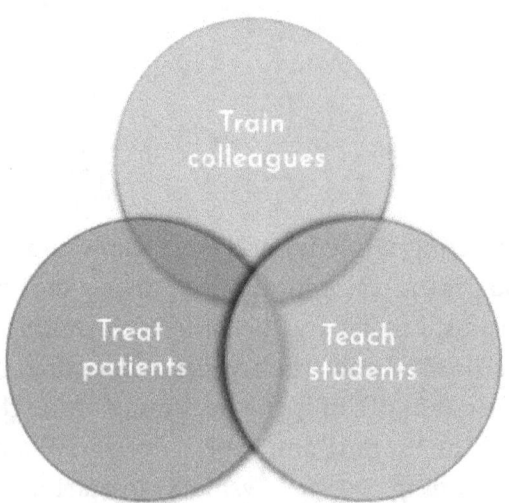

The rest of this chapter features my detailed thoughts and observations on how each of these three Ts can play out for a robust and worthwhile career as a consulting physician.

The First T: Treat Your Patient

Something you'll come across later on, in chapter 25 "Dr. Taha's 11 Keys to Success," is communication. Not only in building yourself a successful career, but ensuring that your patient interactions are also as optimal as possible, your ability to communicate well is key. Communicating doesn't just refer to your ability to talk to patients. Yes, that's important, but it's much more than that. As I see it, a doctor with effective communication builds a rapport with their patients, practices active listening with them, knows how to ask effective questions, can explain things appropriately, practices discretion, and can effectively communicate with a patient's family. Let's look into these aspects in more detail, so you can become a great communicator with your patients.

Rapport

As you know from your time in medical school and from your residency, it is demanding work being a consulting physician. It's not uncommon that doctors feel tired and pressured to meet the demands of the job. Because of this, our patients can assume from our demeanor that we are not listening to them or explaining things to them thoroughly. That we aren't really open and available. Basically, many patients consider doctors lousy communicators.

I can see where patients are coming from with this complaint. My solution is to actively and purposefully build rapport with each patient. Even though it might seem extra work and outside our job description to make a patient feel like we have a connection, in fact, it can make all the difference in them being open and honest with us and with them taking our recommendations and acting on them. Think about it—it makes sense. If you think someone is in a rush and feeling tense, would you really want to share with them the whole story about your breathing issue? Would you really trust their advice if you don't think they listened to you in the first place?

To build rapport, this is what I recommend you do. Before entering the room, take a deep breath and let go of whatever previous interactions or worries that have been buzzing around your mind. You might even want to have a go-to phrase that you say aloud to yourself to "seal" this letting-go: "That was then and this is now," "I'm taking things in stride and living in the present." Something like that, to make it more concrete the letting go. If you are particularly stressed and amped, it could be a good idea to take more than twenty seconds to return to your present self and let go. You might need to drink a cup of tea or take a look out the window at the horizon to get some perspective and some distance. The point is to gain some self-awareness and dislodge any clutter that has be plaguing your mind. When you make it a habit, it becomes easier too.

When you are present and settled, that's when you enter the patient's room. If you haven't met the person before, acknowledge that. Introduce yourself, "Hello. My name is … ." You could standardize your first-time meeting with a patient by including rapport-building comments. Similarly, you could standardize your whole method for building rapport. It should certainly involve eye contact and smiling. It might also involve taking a seat (rather than standing which can look like you are ready to exit) and asking a question (from a set of five you have on hand).

Mirroring another person's posture, stance, tone of voice, and language is another way to build rapport—as long as it is subtle.

When you come across as attentive and friendly, even if it adds another two minutes to your visit, it will pay dividends in the quality of service you can provide to them. They will relax and start to trust you, both of which are key in helping them.

Active Listening

After you build rapport and it's time to get down to business—the reason for the visit—that first minute you give the patient to explain themselves is important. Let them speak. Don't interrupt them. This allows them to feel listened to and respected. Plus, they might divulge some useful information without even exactly realizing it.

Active listening is multifaceted. There's both what they are saying and the undertones—the emotional element behind what they are saying. For most people, being sick, feeling weak, being in pain, and visiting the doctor is not the joy of their life. It can be scary, difficult, and stressful. When you summarize back to the person what you heard them articulate to you—also a useful strategy not only to show you were listening to them but to make sure what you heard is accurate—you could add in your recognition of the emotional toll it is taking on them. For example, "Tell me if this is correct—you are missing work today because of a sudden pain in your left ear. It happened last night and you expected it to go away, but it didn't. I imagine this is both difficult and stressful for you, so let's figure it out. First, tell me if I'm understanding you correctly." Doing this demonstrates your empathy for their situation. And that they aren't just another case for you to check off the list for the day.

Also, believe it or not—it is more efficient for you to provide an empathetic summary to them, where they confirm or correct your summary, than if you don't. When you don't confirm with a summary, patients often don't feel heard and will repeat their story in an attempt to get recognition. This can take additional time.

Effective Questioning

While I acknowledge that as doctors we are like sleuths, trying to get to bottom of a mystery, it can be ineffective to shower a series of questions on a patient. They can feel interrogated, particularly if it is yes-or-no questions you are peppering them with. Plus, you might not be eliciting the full information and instead letting your assumptions take the lead.

Start your questioning with open-ended questions. Think—who? What? When? Where? How? You will get a more complete response that will help you build important background. From there, you can dig down to more specific and closed questions to uncover red flags or rule out particular diseases, viruses, or other conditions. Don't just jump to a conclusion. Keep your mind open when assessing.

Be wary of asking leading questions, this means questions where you point the respondee to the answer you want in the way you ask the question. For instance, this is a leading question, "You don't have a headache, do you?" To please you or not argue, they might simply take your lead and say no even if it isn't true.

You could even ask them their take on what's going on. Finding out their perspective on, for example, why they believe their knee hurts, could reveal something from their health background that relates to their symptoms that help you a lot.

As already stated, visiting the doctor is scary and stressful for people, so allowing them to articulate their greatest worry is a way to offer them assurance. For example, "When you think about your earache, is there anything in particular that concerns you? Do you have any lingering questions I could address?" From here, they may reveal a worst-case scenario—for example, that they are on their way to losing their hearing like what happened to their uncle—that you can quickly dispel.

Effective Explaining

Incredibly, research found that patients typically forget 40% to 80% of the medical information we provide them. Immediately. How can we remedy this? One way is to tailor our responses to the specific questions the patients ask. We could also write down or do an audio recording of the information we are providing them. We should avoid speaking at length. Instead, we should deliver parcels of information, with pauses in between, in which we check in with the patient to see if they understand or have questions.

Another option is to ask the patient to do for you what you did for them at the start of the consultation. To provide you with a summary of what they understand you've told them. This is a great way to determine what they understood, misunderstood, and what they didn't take in. Then you can provide clarity and add on other important points—and again ask them to summarize their new understanding.

Also, if possible provide them with written information like pamphlets or leaflets or send them to a website that you find valuable.

Because patients typically want to be involved in their healthcare decisions and want to know more, it is critical that you work out a way to ensure that they are taking in the correct information from your words and that they have other options for gathering credible information. The more a patient understands about their health situation, the more responsibility they can take on to improve it, which is what we as doctors are aiming for.

Discretion

Particularly on an open ward of a hospital, it can be tricky to keep your patient interaction private. With only curtains affording you privacy, depending on the level of sensitivity of the information you are going to provide, it could be a good idea to find a closed-door space to talk to someone. Something else to consider is your own mobile phone—you don't want it interrupting you with pings or even ringing when you are talking to a patient, especially if you are delivering troubling or bad news. Be sensitive to the person's privacy needs and also their need to feel respected.

Communicating with Family

It isn't uncommon that a consulting physician must speak to the family of a patient to let them know what's going on with the patient. Always remember to take into account the patient's right and the privacy laws of your jurisdiction, even when speaking with a family member.

Remember that your first duty is to the patient—and not to their family. While you may think you are being helpful by informing the family about what's going on with the patient, you could very well be wrong. For this reason, get express permission from the patient about speaking to their family, whether it be a conversation in person or over the phone. Also, determine with the patient what you will and won't discuss with the family. For example, perhaps the patient's past medical history comes into play with their current situation. That past medical history could be sensitive and the patient might have never shared it with family members. They might not want you to discuss that. The point is to get consent from patients on whether or not you can speak to their families and what you are allowed to disclose.

Another helpful option is to try to have a discussion with family members in the presence of the patient. This way, the patient is aware of exactly what you say. This can avoid miscommunication and misinterpretations later on, on either the family's or the patient's part.

You want the patient to know you are being frank and open with them and not telling your family a different story.

Expect at some point that a family member will ask you to withhold key information from a patient, especially if it's about a condition that is untreatable or very serious. It is your duty to be upfront with the family about your obligations to the patient first and foremost. Your patient must be informed of their condition. It is part of your job. Be clear with the family on this. It might be tempting to soft-peddle and not fully disclose to the family that you will tell the patient everything. You must be upfront and clear. Although the family could make a good argument that it is detrimental to the patient's psyche to hear the truth, if the patient is deemed competent, you must disclose the truth to them.

When there is a large family, it can be easier and less confusing for you to ask that one or two of them serve as your point of contact. It is common for doctors to make this a practice to save time and avoid confusion.

The Second T: Teach Students

Among the parts of the Hippocratic Oath is to teach medical trainees: "I will respect the hard-won scientific gains of those physicians in whose steps I walk, and gladly share such knowledge as is mine with those who are to follow." It is a tradition for doctors to teach medical students and colleagues. However, it can be very challenging to be an effective teacher, especially when you have so many competing demands. It isn't uncommon for doctors to find themselves in this situation.

You like teaching new interns, registrars/residents, and medical school students, but you find that you are expected to do more and more teaching of greater numbers of trainees and the paperwork that goes along with it is getting more complicated and extensive. You realize that many of your colleagues appear to be great teachers. You wonder how they got so good, what they are doing, and how you can be as effective as they are while continuing to manage your regular medical work.

Not surprisingly, the performance of your students and trainees will correlate with your teaching abilities. Good doctor teachers are not just good doctors, meaning good at practicing medicine, they are also good at teaching their students and trainees how to practice medicine. Plus, they are good supervisors. You can be a good doctor but a lousy teacher. You can be a mediocre doctor and a good teacher (though probably not effective). To be effective you must be both a good doctor and a good teacher and supervisor. Yes, this is a lot, especially considering you are already working so hard.

An effective medical doctor and teacher encompasses all of the following:

- They act as a good medical doctor role model—they are competent, professional, knowledgeable, and caring.
- They are a skilled supervisor—they know how to give feedback, involve trainees in clinical care, and give direction in patient care when it is required.
- They provide their students and trainees with support—caring, mentoring, providing career advice, and showing an interest.
- They are solid teachers—motivating, planning, identifying what students and trainees need to learn and how to go about filling in those gaps.

Similar to what I was talking about previously, in terms of building a rapport with your patient in order to be an effective doctor, you also must nurture an interpersonal relationship with your students in order for your teaching to be effective. It might sound too soft or touchy-feely, but when you show your students and trainees that you care about them and their learning, when they are aware of your consideration of them, they will respond better to your teaching.

If you are teaching junior doctors, residents, or registrars, and if they are under your charge, it means that they will actually be taking on patients and caring for them. It is only natural that they will make mistakes at times and make decisions that aren't that great.

As their teacher, you need to anticipate this and do your best to keep mistakes to a minimum. And when they do make a mistake, help them to learn from their mistake. Facilitate that learning rather than shaming them or blaming them.

What are the typical challenges you'll face?

The biggest challenge is not enough time. Because you'll have a greater amount of work to undertake for both patients and administration, the amount of time available to be a good teacher will never feel like enough. Plus, you'll find that there are not very many patients you can use with your medical students, that your patients are staying in the hospital for too short a time to be helpful cases, and the patients that are staying longer are incredibly sick such that their cases are too complex to work with.

Another major challenge is the fact that teaching itself requires a different skillset than does practicing medicine. And it isn't likely you'll be trained in the art of teaching. Figuring out your students' competence levels, figuring out how to motivate your students, giving them feedback that is helpful, teaching students who are at multiple levels at the same time (all while dealing with doing your regular job) falls under the scope of teaching and will likely be new to you, as most doctors have never been taught how to teach, supervise, or assess students.

With all the effort you put in to do your best at teaching, you will be criticized for not being good enough. For some doctor teachers, this criticism is merited. Research shows that some medical doctor teachers humiliate their students and are sarcastic, or else the quality of there teaching is unpredictable and changing day by day without enough supervision, feedback, and assessment. Many hospitals have been advised that their doctor teachers need teacher training themselves.

It is getting harder and harder for rising doctors to attain the level of expertise needed to practice as consulting physicians. It is imperative that we consulting physicians put in the effort to teach our students effectively, even in the face of all the other challenges. Being an effective teacher means that you give your students feedback on their work. You work with them to identify their gaps and to make goals to fill them. You give regular assessments and discuss the results with them. You make a learning plan with them as well. Yes, all this requires time and effort, but it's what makes teaching effective, rewarding, and enjoyable, both for your students and for you.

What else? Realize too that not all students learn in the same way, so you may need to adjust your style to accommodate different learning needs. Be ready to evaluate your own teaching. Be ready to learn new methods and to evaluate the effectiveness of your various teaching methods. Get feedback on your teaching as well. Just like being a medical doctor, teaching is something you get better at. It's not set in stone.

For Resident/Registrar Doctors Also Teaching Medical Students

As a resident/registrar, you will probably be expected to train or teach medical students in some capacity. Rather than seeing this as another drag on your time, I challenge you to see it as a unique opportunity that you can seize. Why? Because you are in a special position—more than a medical student but not yet a consulting physician. Because you exist between these two worlds, you are in a great position to relate to what medical students are going through. You have a fresh memory of where they are at, what their needs are, and how important it is for someone in a more senior position—which you are to them—to show them respect, to motivate and inspire them, and to teach them, perhaps in the way that you wish your resident/registrar had taught you. What I aim to provide in this article is advice specifically for residents/registrars who have been charged with teaching medical school students and are at the same time trainees themselves. Yes, it's a lot of work, but hopefully, my advice will help you manage your responsibilities more easily.

As mentioned earlier in this chapter, a doctor isn't naturally or automatically a good teacher. But, it's expected of doctors to teach and support rising doctors. When you are undergoing a strenuous residency program yourself—when you are already expected to master the processes of diseases, when you are stressed with medical decision making with real patients, and when you are already struggling to speak to patients in the language that they, the patient, can understand—teaching medical students as well can seem like your lowest priority. One way to gain more enthusiasm and motivation around teaching medical students is to take on the perspective that through teaching them, you, yourself will also increase your own knowledge of disease processes and other issues you are expected to master during your residency. Here are some more recommendations for turning teaching medical students into an opportunity rather than a burden.

Ground Rules

From the start establish some ground rules with the medical student. This is true whether you'll be interacting with the student for just a day or a few weeks. The first ground rule is simply working out the logistics: when they should arrive, how they should prepare before arriving, when to ask questions, and the appropriate length of time interacting with patients. By establishing these logistical ground rules at the start, both you and the student will more easily get along and make progress together. It is equally important to establish the goal of the medical student during their time with you—what is it they are hoping to learn? Of course, all the while you should show yourself as personable and approachable to them. By putting into effect these ground rules from the start, even if it takes a bit of time, your overall experience as teacher and student will be easier and more satisfying for all parties involved.

Hypotheticals

Just as your trainers and professors have done with you, it is your duty to teach the medical students to become thinkers. A great way of doing this is to create hypotheticals that extrapolate the case of one patient. I'm talking about asking, "What if … ?" Because medical students have a limited knowledge base (which expands with each ensuing training experience), they often approach patients with too narrow of a focus in terms of diagnoses and treatments. Another common situation is that the medical student has an extensive knowledge base but has no experience applying it in real-world situations. They need guidance. To help students in both categories to become thinkers, you can dig into your own knowledge and experience to ask them a "What if ... ?" question, asking what if another symptom presented itself here or what if the exam was different. In this way, based on a single patient encounter, the student can glean even more experience. They have greater opportunities to expand their diagnosis or treatment considerations. They develop themselves as thinkers.

Patience

So many times in this book we have gone back to the incredibly demanding nature of medical training and how it never seems we have enough time. Because of this, it is incredibly important that you practice patience with your medical students and also with your own patients. Good teachers are patient. You already know that as you've likely witnessed or been the victim of an impatient teacher, one who has cut you off or cut short someone else's presentation. Be aware of how easy it is to slip into impatient mode. Purposefully cultivate patience. For example, when a student is speaking to you, allow them to say their complete thought. Don't cut them off. If you ask them a question and they don't immediately respond, wait. Don't rush in with a hint or with the answer. Wait and let them formulate their thoughts. If you need to set a timer to ensure that you give each student three minutes to present their patient, that's three minutes without you interrupting, then do so. Actually, in your ground rules you could establish the expectation of the medical student spending three minutes to present their patient. This time expectation will also help them be prepared, concise, and more efficient.

Key Points

To help your medical students move from simply collecting information, to processing and synthesizing that information, after the medical student presents the patient presentation, you can summarize and say back to them the most important points from their presentation. Doing this demonstrates your thought process and it also allows them to focus on the most important points (as opposed to all the points) when they come to the diagnosis. In medical school students collect a lot of information, but they haven't learned yet how to apply that information. When you parse the information about a patient and iterate back to them what you hear as the most important pieces of information, you are teaching them to go beyond collecting and to start applying. You are teaching them how to process information, which will be key in their moving through the clinical years. By repeating key points and salient facts back to the student, you teach them how to narrow down on the important information to arrive at the best diagnosis. Later on, they will likely remember this when experiencing a similar case.

Feedback

Especially when a medical student makes a mistake, it is important to give them specific feedback early on about what happened. This will help them to avoid such errors, not only when they are with you but also in the future. You don't have to be harsh when you point out an error to them. You can do it kindly and professionally, but it is critical you give them feedback immediately so they have a complete memory and understanding of exactly what they did wrong and how they can correct it. Even if it might make you feel awkward, medical students are grateful for feedback. That's how they improve. If your feedback is positive, then it's acceptable to deliver it in front of a patient or colleague. However, if you have a correction to make, and the feedback is pointing out an error, it's best to do it as soon as possible but also only with them. Not in the presence of anyone else. For some students, it is important to differentiate whether your feedback is intended for their improvement or if it is related to an evaluation. Again, when you make the effort to provide feedback that improves a medical student, and you do so in a kind way, they will look back on you as helpful in making them into a competent doctor.

Don't shrug off the teaching responsibilities simply because it is one task among too many during your residency years. Teaching medical students is valuable and critical, and it can also be rewarding when you put in the effort. Remember to begin by establishing the ground rules. Help them expand their thinking by asking the hypothetical "What if … ?" questions. Be patient. Highlight back to them the key points in their presentations and provide them with immediate feedback, especially if they commit an error. It's only natural that each resident will develop their own style of teaching, but because people learn in a different way, you might have to adjust your style at times. It is likely you are going to be asked to do a lot of teaching during your residency. By applying my recommendations you can transform that teaching experience into something that both you and your students find rewarding.

The Third T: Train Your Colleagues

In the second T, "Teach Students," we already talked about how teaching up-and-coming doctors was a longtime expectation of practicing doctors. Even still, it seems that consulting physicians need additional support to become better teachers, trainers, and mentors to those studying medicine. In this third T "Train Your Colleagues," I'm going to write specifically about considerations for doctors to become better quality teachers for residents training under them.

While you probably remember your residency years as being challenging and exhausting times, it is likely that what current residents are experiencing is even more so. The reason is due to changes in residency training, the greater amount of knowledge and skills they are expected to master, the massive costs of medical school and training, and the decrease in the available time with faculty because of the greater demands in terms of residents' academic, clinical, and research. These new demands require that they learn new and complex approaches: competency-based assessments, simulations, and online courses and resources. I'm sharing this with you so that you have some kind of understanding of what residents are going through.

As we already know, for residents to bridge the gap between the medical knowledge they've spent years accumulating and the art of applying that knowledge with patients via medical practice, faculty are key. The resident will look at all the faculty as role models, seeking information, guidance, and mentoring. Faculty members must remember that all residents hold them up as role models. They mustn't underestimate the impact they are having. For these reasons, faculty should make sure to exhibit the characteristics of availability, accessibility, professionalism, accountability, and congeniality with residents. When faculty are teaching residents, they must make their teaching a priority, they must be willing to teach and to adjust their style of teaching to accommodate their students' needs, and they must remain committed to the full length of the teaching project. As mentors, the faculty should make sure to make time for residents and show interest in them. As role models to residents, faculty should make an effort to participate in community-minded activities. In order to support faculty being the most effective for residents, institutions should make the effort to compensate faculty members for their efforts, to make research opportunities available to faculty, to recognize outstanding faculty, and to do all they can to have high faculty retention rates.

While education is obviously the purpose of residency, it can sometimes seem that the specialty training required by residents and the way it is organized is so challenging that it is almost impossible for residents to achieve the education they are supposed to be getting. There is so much for residents to learn—so many settings, curriculum, and techniques. And even with all these challenges, residents along with faculty members are expected to provide optimal patient care.

I argue that in order for a residency program to deliver a high quality of education to residents/registrars there are certain characteristics that must be exhibited. Active teaching, meaning bedside teaching, must happen during patient care in every setting. The curriculum should have distinct goals and objectives. The resident should encounter a variety of patients, therapeutic modalities, pathologies, and practice settings. The curriculum should be relevant both to clinical practice and to exams.

What I mean by that is during residency, the education provided should prepare residents/registrars for in-service, boards, and post-residency practice (in-service exams are preparation for the board exams, and specialty board exams test knowledge required for post-residency practice in the given specialty).

Over the years of residency, the residents/registrars should experience ever-increasing levels of responsibility with appropriate supervision at each given level. There should be regularly scheduled morbidity and mortality conferences. Supervisors should routinely assess residents'/registrars' proficiency and competency in clinical skills.

There are a number of areas residents/registrars should be given guidance in, perhaps in the form of professional development sessions. In no particular order, these areas include professionalism, communication skills, personal standards and ethics, errors (how to avoid and handle errors), practice management, advocacy issues, medico-legal issues, finding and using leadership opportunities, contracts and negotiation, improving morale, quality assurance, preparation for education beyond residency training, research skills, critical thinking skills, evidence-based medicine, hospital infrastructure, CV and job interview preparation, teaching skills, computers and informatics, medical technology practice management, medical procedure skills, resource conservation, and documentation (informed consent, medical records, coding, etc.).

I also advocate a multi-disciplinary approach to teaching throughout training. And it would be valuable that departmental and hospital committees involved with resident training, resident education and patient care have resident representatives on them.

As you already know I am a person who likes to push the envelope, expand my own horizons, and increase my learning, so I'm going to share with you an endeavor that exists outside the realm of medicine. Chapter 23 describes how I came to be operating in a kitchen!

Chapter 23
Operating in a Kitchen

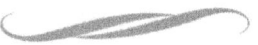

ecause the ongoing themes of this book entail grabbing the
bull by the horns and embarking on new adventures to expand
your horizons as an aspiring, studying, training, and/or already
consulting physician and doing a lot of preplanning and connecting with
mentors to make it all possible, in this chapter I offer a variation on that
theme. This variation is parallel to our book's main theme of expanding
your medical horizons (and doing a lot of planning), but it is outside of
the realm of medicine. In this chapter we enter the realm of business
and gastronomy, namely oriental food in a chic Zürich eatery. Now that
I've piqued your interest and probably got your tastebuds watering, let's
delve in!

Mohamed Khalil Ali, one of my friends for the last ten years since I
came to Switzerland, is an outstanding cook. Before I left for Australia,
he told me, "I've been working in a big Lebanese chain of restaurants for
the past five years, and now it's time to move on. I want to open my own
restaurant. If you'd be interested, I'd love for you to be a partner in my
new restaurant."

Because of all the time, energy, and financial stress my family and
I were under in order to make the yearlong fellowship in Australia
happen, I let Mohamed know that at that time, I wasn't prepared to join
him. However, I added, "Maybe after Australia."

When I returned to Switzerland from Australia, Mohamed again asked, "So now that you are back, what do you think about partnering to start a restaurant?"

While I had no experience with cooking, restaurants, or even businesses, something I did know about was the importance of consulting with mentors and doing a lot of planning. Actually, embarking upon this restaurant start-up with Mohamed reminded me a lot of what it's like to engage in clinical research. Once I realized this, I was able to work with Mohamed and our restaurant business using this similarity as my guide. Let's look at the similarities.

Parallels Between Clinical Research and Business

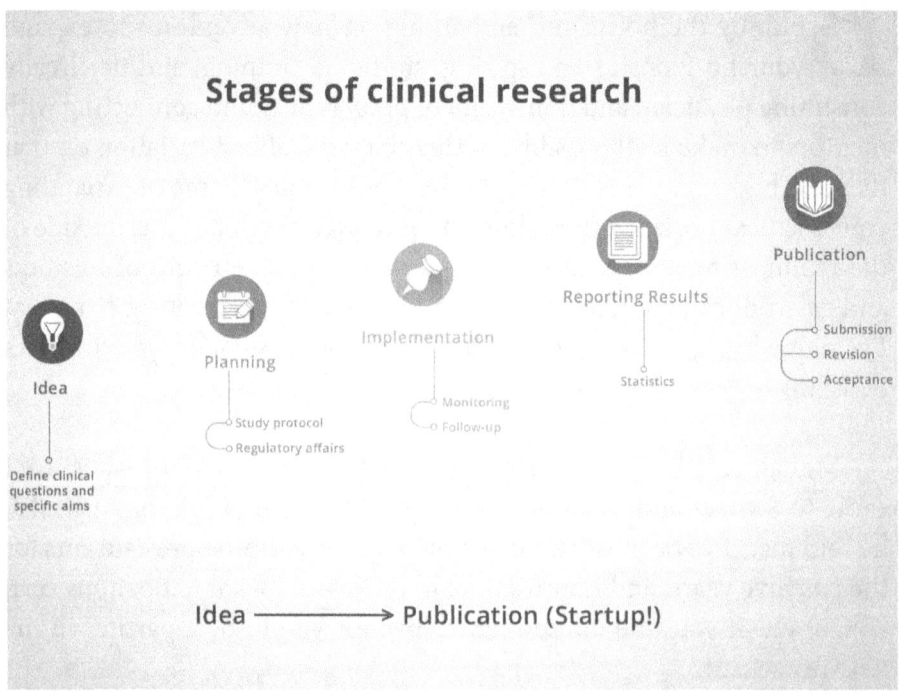

Conducting a clinical research study and starting up a business have many parallels. First, both start with an idea. However, for both, a vague idea isn't enough. You can't get approval or funding based on an idea alone. Lots of parameters must be mapped out and articulated first. In clinical research you may start with a general idea, but from there you must define your clinical question and specific aims for the study. In business, when you have an idea, you still have to determine your target clientele, the business's specific aim, and the particular value your business will add to the market. For both, you start questioning your idea at the very first step to narrow it and shape it.

After that, in both research and business, the next step is planning. In research, the planning is called a study protocol and in business it is called a business plan. This is when you go through the planning and the numbers to determine whether it is it feasible or not to pursue the clinical research and/or business idea.

After finishing the second step, if you decide to continue, then you move to step three, which is implementation. For a business, implementation is when you monitor its expected performance, follow up on meetings, and get the finances and accounting in order. For a clinical research study implementation is similar. It's when you are recruiting patients, determining whether you have enough cases and whether followups are working.

Step four is the reporting. For a study, it is where you write up and determine the results and analyze them. For a business, it is where you do the analysis, going deep into the numbers, to determine profits, costs, and next steps.

Finally, for both it is about "going public," so to speak. For a research study, that means getting published. For a business start-up, it is the launching of the real business or product. With both a study and a business, it could take years of study and planning before actually launching.

Sim-Sim

When Mohamed and I started our restaurant business project, we started with step one as outlined above. We addressed the questions: "What is our mission? What is our value proposal? Why are we different?"

Next, we made a business plan and created all the value on the website, IT, and such. Again, there were many areas that I didn't know much about or that were completely new to me, so to navigate these unknowns we sought out good mentors, people who have been there before, and we asked for their help.

After six months of research and planning, Mohamed and I finally opened the restaurant, Sim-Sim Restaurant (www.sim-sim.ch). I was responsible for planning and determining the global concept. Mohamed takes the technical part of cooking and running the restaurant itself. It was Mohamed's dream and as his friend I supported him to make it come true.

As of September 2019 we're one year in, and I'm pleased to report that Sim-Sim is working very well. So far, we've had tons of visits to our restaurant's webpage. Our average review as given on various review sites is five stars. We're getting more and more customers every day. Mohamed is living his dream and enjoying the satisfaction of his clientele.

Sim-Sim and You

My aim in telling you about Sim-Sim is to provide you yet another example of the importance of keeping your head up and supporting your family, friends, and mentees, even when you are incredibly busy with your medical studies or medical career. Also, Sim-Sim illustrates, via another avenue, the importance of planning and finding good mentors to support you so that you can better predict and overcome the many challenges and unknowns that will appear in your pursuit of an international fellowship, observership, or some other fantastic opportunity you look to do.

I write this again because it is just so helpful: consider MY-FELLOWSHIP, a multifaceted opportunity that lays out the aspects of the planning you'll need to consider and provides the mentors to help you navigate the process when you pursue fellowship and observership opportunities. If you are starting your career in a certain specialty or if you're looking to learn a new technique, a new operation, or a new research project, MY-FELLOWSHIP offers the insights, resources, and mentors for you to make it happen. Don't reinvent the wheel. Make use of the resources MY-FELLOWSHIP offers. If you have done an observership, fellowship, or want to offer a mentorship, observership, or fellowship, I urge you to go to www.myfellowship.com and share your experience.

I agree that it might seem hard to leave your comfort zone and start something new—such as an international fellowship or observership—but the learning, mentors, and travel experience you'll engage with make it worth it. Plus, MY-FELLOWSHIP provides so much assistance that deciding where to apply and applying (plus sorting out the other requirements after you are accepted) is very doable. You don't have any excuses not to expand your horizons!

Speaking of MY-FELLOWSHIP, chapter 24 details the growth journey of the platform, from its inception as an idea to how I envision its future playing out, a future that should help doctors and patients the world over.

Chapter 24

Let's Change the World Together: MY-FELLOWSHIP

Let's take a look at the story of www.myfellowship.com, so you can follow the steps I took to bring this seed of an idea to fruition. Some of this information I've given earlier in the book, but here in this chapter I'm putting it together to give you the complete story. You'll learn about the stakeholders I approached for feedback on my ideas, the survey I sent out to get feedback from a greater pool of stakeholders, the three benefits everyone identified for doing a fellowship, as well as the four biggest problems they cited around finding fellowships, problems that MY-FELLOWSHIP offers solutions to.

As noted in chapter 16, it was during my fellowship in Australia that I met several fellows who were frustrated with their fellowship experience. They said it wasn't what they'd expected when they applied and got accepted. I wondered if the problem wasn't the fellowships they were doing, but that they hadn't had the complete information to make an informed decision. It was my interactions with these dissatisfied fellows in combination with the arduous multi-stepped process I had to go through (1) to apply to fellowships and then once accepted (2) to get the paperwork completed to make the fellowships happen that sparked the idea for the MY-FELLOWSHIP platform.

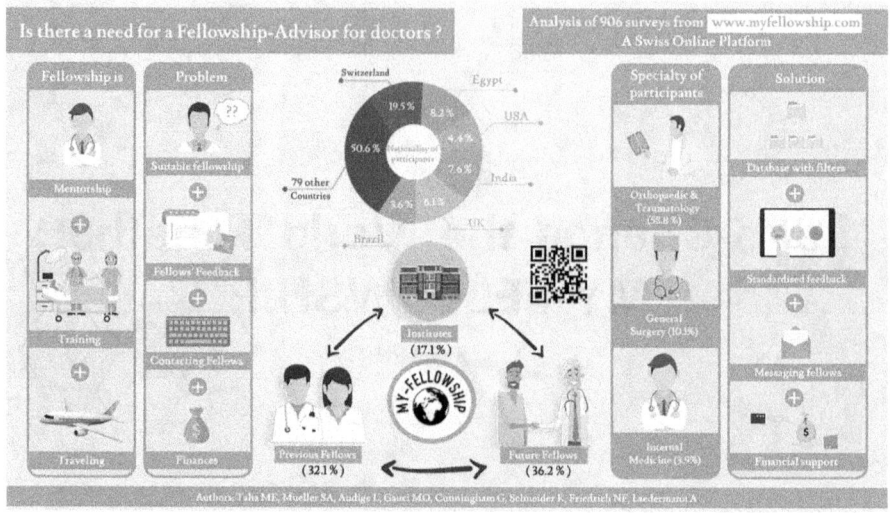

Once I got the idea for the platform, I decided to speak to stakeholders, i.e., mentors, to see if they thought the idea for the MY-FELLOWSHIP platform was worthy of pursuing further. These mentor stakeholders I divide into three categories: (1) fellowship providers, (2) past fellows, and (3) future fellows.

Mentors: Fellowship Providers

When I had the idea of starting the MY-FELLOWSHIP platform, my next move was to speak to some mentors. These were people who had done fellowships themselves and who currently were fellowship providers. I approached them to pitch my idea. I explained the problems and how I saw the platform as offering solutions. I asked for their opinion, feedback, and such. Interestingly, these fellowship provider mentors agreed that they thought the platform was a very good idea. They were interested in the project.

Benefits for fellowship providers:

- Join our database of worldwide fellowships
- Add, edit, manage, and update their fellowship/s 24/7
- Receive unbiased feedback from previous fellows on the platform (can be deactivated)

- Access and contact doctors and researchers looking for fellowships
- Connect with previous fellows

Mentors: Fellows, Past and Future

After getting positive feedback from fellowship providers, I approached other consulting physicians, who, like me, had done fellowships. Again, I talked to them about what I saw as problems pursuing fellowships and how I saw the MY-FELLOWSHIP platform as offering solutions. I asked them for their input, ideas, opinions, and feedback. Similar to the fellowship providers, whom I first approached, this group of previous fellows also agreed that the platform was a good idea. Many of them particularly appreciated that the platform would connect aspiring fellows to mentors, mentors in terms of fellowship providers and previous fellows.

Next, I spoke to aspiring fellows and residents/registrars who someday would want to pursue fellowships and observerships. Upon asking them, "What do you think of such a project?" they responded enthusiastically, "That would be a great help for us to find fellowships!" And so that was the very first phase.

Because I wanted feedback from an even larger segment of people, I came up with the idea of doing a survey. I launched a landing page pitching my idea, telling people what I was thinking about. Then I created an online survey asking, "What problems do you have with fellowships? How can we solve them?" The survey listed examples where respondents could choose from a list of problems and solutions. Also, people had the option to write in their own ideas. We offered this survey on the website.

We launched the site at the beginning of December, announcing it at an orthopedics conference in Switzerland, where people from all over the world had gathered together. Within five months the MY-FELLOWSHIP site had about 9,000 visits. We received back 906 surveys from people in 85 countries. From the results, we were able to identify three main benefits of a fellowship—mentorship, training, and traveling—and we were able to identify the four main problems that people doing, or looking to do, fellowships recommended that the MY-FELLOWSHIP site address:

1. Finding relevant fellowships
2. Getting feedback from previous fellows about fellowships
3. Contacting previous fellows to learn more
4. Financing a fellowship

Let's look at those two aspects: the three parts of a fellowship and then the four problems survey respondents hoped MY-FELLOWSHIP would address.

The Three Parts of a Fellowship: Mentorship, Training, Traveling

The benefits of a fellowship can be sorted into three main categories: mentorship, training, and traveling. The mentorship aspect comes into play when you meet the leader or advisor of the fellowship program. The training is the medical work you are observing, assisting with, and doing yourself. The third aspect is traveling because it is typical that in a fellowship you go to a new place, either a new place in your own country or to a totally different country. As already discussed in this book, I'm calling the three benefits of doing a fellowship, the "fellowship triangle."

The Four Problems Around Fellowships and MY-FELLOWSHIP's Solutions

1 - Finding Relevant Fellowships

This is the very first challenge. If you go to the internet and type "fellowship" into Google, you get around 170 million results. How are you going to choose one fellowship out of 170 million? There is so much irrelevant information out there. Plus the word "fellowship" itself can have many different meanings. So, the very first problem we identified was how to find suitable fellowships. Aspiring fellows need a central location where a multitude of fellowships are featured. MY-FELLOWSHIP aims to be this central location.

MY-FELLOWSHIP features a database, with different filters, where participants can filter each fellowship according to their needs, such as specialty, subspecialty, location, country, city, language, paid/not paid, and financial support/no financial support. You can filter all of this with a couple of clicks to find fellowships suitable for you.

2 - Feedback on Those Fellowships

The next problem is getting feedback about any given fellowship. I'm talking about a review-feedback system like at TripAdvisor, Airbnb, Yelp, and such. Before visiting a restaurant or choosing a place to stay, you can go to one of these sites to read about it beforehand. You can read about the personal experiences of others who have done it before you to understand the pros and cons. When you plan a holiday for one week, then you spend time to check reviews of the hotels and restaurants. And that's only for one week. For a fellowship, you're going to spend one year in a foreign country with somebody as a mentor whom you've never met before. It is a tough decision and you need a lot of information to decide to put in the big effort to apply to it, and if you are accepted, you need full information to decide to commit to it. Currently, MY-FELLOWSHIP features plenty of fellowships, added from previous fellows or fellowship providers, as well as reviews of those fellowships, so that potential applicants can access the nitty-gritty feedback from previous fellows to help make the most informed decisions.

We developed a standardized feedback system where a fellowship is broken down into categories, e.g., mentorship with the training, clinical research, hands-on training, teaching, etc. Previous fellows then provide feedback about these aspects of the fellowship. In turn, this multi-faceted feedback should help you determine whether a fellowship is suitable.

3 - Contacting Previous Fellows to Learn More

Furthermore, you might need to contact a fellow who has been there before and given feedback to discuss further details with them. For example, if you've been accepted, you might want to ask them any of the following questions: where do I find an apartment? Can my spouse and kids go with me? Is there a school? Are there any tricks or tips for getting a visa? You will have hundreds of questions about living in the new country, and many of these questions won't be directly related to the fellowship's medical training and the fellowship itself, but they are very significant. MY-FELLOWSHIP offers you access to previous fellows, so you can get answers to your many questions.

Benefits for previous fellows:

- Expand your network to fellowship-trained surgeons around the world
- Help fellowship providers and future fellows
- Influence the careers of your colleagues
- Contribute to the community by adding a fellowship
- Connect to and mentor future fellows

4 - Financial Support

The fourth important problem, which almost everyone mentioned, is finding financial support to go abroad and do your fellowship. Let's say you find a suitable fellowship, you get accepted, and to do it you need financial support, then you can apply to MY-FELLOWSHIP to get that financial support. We connect fellows to sponsors so that fellows can get their fellowships sponsored.

MY-FELLOWSHIP Challenge

If you are a future fellow looking for a fellowship, I challenge you to go to the platform, www.myfellowship.com, and search for suitable fellowships. Input your filters to find five fellowships suitable for you.

If you are a previous fellow, I ask that you go to the site, www. myfellowship.com, and give you feedback about that fellowship so that (1) future fellows can profit from your experience and (2) you can mentor new fellows.

If you are a fellowship provider, please go to the platform, www. myfellowship.com, and add your fellowship to the MY-FELLOWSHIP database. We invite you to join us.

In collaboration with the VSAO-Basel (Association of Swiss Residents and Consultants) we launched MY-FELLOWSHIP which is the world's first free fellowships encyclopedia from doctors and researchers that is built from the ground up according to their needs. If you would like to know more about how MY-FELLOWSHIP can help your medical career or what you can do to contribute, please visit us at www.myfellowship. com.

As this book is about to come to a close, the next chapter (the chapter before the final one) presents the 11 variables that I think a person must consider to be successful in their endeavors. I call these "Dr. Taha's 11 Keys to Success."

All revenue generated from this book will be donated to the community platform: www.myfellowship.com

Future Is Yours

Chapter 25

Dr. Taha's 11 Keys to Success

W hen looking through my past experiences and considering, "What did and what didn't work out? And if something worked out, why did it work?" I've come up with 11 aspects that play a big role in the success or lack of success. As I want you to succeed in your medical studies, consultancy, and in pursuing international fellowships and observerships, please consider these 11 aspects in these major endeavors. These are our keys to success.

1—Quality

For whatever product or service you are providing, it needs to be of the highest quality possible. In order to succeed today, your competition isn't based solely in your neighborhood, city, region, or country. Today, it's a worldwide market. Globalization is affecting all of us. The way to differentiate yourself is through the high quality of the product or service you offer. When you do your best to offer the highest quality possible, you can successfully compete everywhere, worldwide and locally.

2—Time

Time is the most precious asset you have because once time goes, it never comes back again. If you want to succeed, you have to appreciate your time and try to be meticulous in how you invest your time.

Be deliberate in deciding how you'll spend each minute and hour of each day.

To improve your use of time consider how to delegate. You cannot do everything yourself. Either you don't have the expertise or the time. Remember, if you delegate a task and even pay someone else to do it, you will save yourself hours and hours. In this way, you gain hours and hours. Delegation is often a great investment.

3—Passion

When you start a project or a career, first you must keep in mind your passion. What are you passionate about? What makes you happy? If you're trying to decide what to do with your studies or career, then start with what you are passionate about. You want your lifelong work and activities to be fun, so go and find your "why."

If you are in the medical field and making a decision about your specialty or subspecialty, again, ask yourself, what is the thing you're passionate about? Don't concentrate on salary. Instead, ask yourself, "What would I love to do?" Once you are passionate about something, and you like it, then you'll be much more productive at it. You can provide much more added value when you choose a specialty you love than if you pick one just because it's, say, a family tradition. Follow your passion.

4—Love

Start by loving yourself because if you don't love yourself, it will be hard for others to love you. Stop beating yourself up for everything that hasn't worked out for you. Start appreciating all of the other things you have achieved in your life. Love yourself, and love the people you serve and the people around you. That's why it's important to do something you are passionate about because then you're passionate also about the people around you—your team—and the people you serve as well—your patients.

Unfortunately, there is a big percentage of people doing jobs that they don't like. They are just doing it because it's a job and it gives them some money. So just by the fact that you love your patients, colleagues, and staff, and you love what you do, then you are going to excel.

5—Your Team

It is incredibly important to have a good team. If you look at the statistics, you will see that among the top reasons start-ups fail is the team. If you choose the wrong team, they will take you down. If you have a good team to support and help you, then they will improve you. You will support one another so that the whole team, and your patients as well, succeed. Because you cannot be an expert in every field, your team can be composed of a variety of experts to offer a range of services to patients and to support one another through everyone's range of expertise.

Put in the effort to join or create a good team, with a range of expertise, who will support one another. Your daily work experience and your whole career will benefit.

6—Communication

I find that one of the important things in work and life is communication. Even communication with yourself. You have to communicate with yourself, "What is my priority? What do I want to do? How am I going to achieve it?" After you communicate it with yourself, then you could communicate it to your team so that everybody is updated and on the same level, thinking, "That's our goal [or mission or vision, etc.]." Most problems come from miscommunication and people not being clear about a message or what they really want. So, find clarity in yourself, and then communicate it clearly with others. Also, be sure to communicate clearly with your patients.

7—Stop Loss

"Stop loss" refers to knowing when to stop in order to limit your losses. When you start a project or a journey, you have a plan, and if it doesn't work, you also have an exit strategy. This way, you can curb your losses before they get too big. Good stop loss plans entail pre-determining the factors that, if they play out, you know you must make your exit from whatever project or plan you are pursuing. Without these stop loss plans in place, you might continue pursuing something that isn't worth it and end up losing a great amount of time, money, energy, or something else that's valuable.

Creating an exit plan and defining the parameters that will determine if, or when, it is necessary to exit a situation are incredibly important to establish from the start. Be sure to stop if those parameters come into play.

8—Selling Before Building

Selling before building. Before pursuing a new project, you must determine beforehand whether or not there is a need for it. For example, if you have an idea for some kind of project or research at your hospital, be sure that before you enact your project, you ask people around you. You do research, you survey people, you send out feedback forms in order to determine whether or not it's a valuable project. It's good to research first, test your idea, and sell your idea before "building" that product or service, before investing time and money in that project. Pitch your idea first and see if there's a need for it before you start building it.

9—Feedback

Enact a feedback system that will allow your patients, clients, colleagues, and partners to give you feedback, so you can improve your service or product. If you have no feedback system, then you could keep making the same mistakes and not know it. It's important to have a system which gives your patients or clients a chance to give you ideas on how to improve, change, develop, and evolve. Maybe what you are doing now is pretty good, but in two years it's not any more attractive because you haven't evolved but your competition has. You need to adjust too, and a feedback system helps you to stay relevant as you move forward.

10—The Game of Life

Recognize life as a game. Then, play to win. If you don't win, you play again and try to win. Each project is like a game and you go in and try to do your best, giving it 100% to win, but then if you lose, it's not the end. It's just time to play another game and play again and try to win. There's no reason to stop or to not keep trying. You always play again, and you try to win.

11—Leverage and Flexibility

You can have much more influence if you are working with different people rather than if you are working alone. Leverage your services (or products) with others who do something similar and be flexible and join up with people who do something different. In this way, you build a robust team that can offer a greater number of services or a higher quality service or who can serve more clients, all of which builds a better, stronger business. Leverage and flexibility will allow you more visibility and influence.

As I'm all about growth and moving forward to expand horizons, grow abilities, and make connections, the final chapter of this book is about just that. Becoming a consulting physician is "only the beginning" of our journey. As long as we are practicing, we must look at increasing our learning and skills. And, of course, MY-FELLOWSHIP aims to help all of us do this!

Chapter 26
It's Only the Beginning

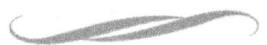

Whatever stage you are at in your medical studies or medical consulting career, it doesn't mean it is the end. Whatever your stage, it's only the beginning of a new challenge. As I see it, we are always meant to be growing, enhancing our skills, increasing our learning, and becoming better. What this means, then, is that once you complete residency and become a physician or once you complete a fellowship and become a fellowship-trained physician, your learning isn't over. Yes, you've completed a significant number of stages in your career journey, but, thankfully, there's more to learn. More to improve. More to enhance.

As physicians, it is imperative that we continue developing our services, we seek feedback from colleagues, staff, and patients in order to help us improve, and that we challenge ourselves by attending conferences, making connections with new experts, and doing more fellowships and observerships. We do not just relax once we become consulting physicians, we continue moving forward.

To inspire you and get you motived for the amazing learning journey that continues even after you become a consultant, let me tell you what I've been up to since September 2017 when I became a consultant. In addition to engaging in the "three Ts" given in chapter 22, I've done eight observerships with doctors in Europe, Canada, and the USA (mentioned in chapter 21). As you are very well aware by now, I founded the MY-

FELLOWSHIP (www.myfellowship.com) platform to make it easier for those of us in the medical world to pursue fellowships and observerships. I am doing clinical and biomechanical research with a focus on the arthroscopic repair of rotator cuff tears and upper limb injuries under the supervision of my mentor PD Dr. Andreas Mueller. Yes, this is a lot, but as I wrote in chapter 25 about the 11 keys to success, it's all possible for me because I am careful about my time management, I am aware of my priorities, and I'm dedicated to my passions. You, too, can do a lot!

The skills you learned during your training and your fellowship do not equate to the end of your learning. Take joy in the fact that you will add and add and add as you go. I invite you to use MY-FELLOWSHIP (www.myfellowship.com) as your go-to tool to increase your skills and abilities. Use this platform to provide a fellowship or observership, share your experience about a fellowship or observership, and/or locate experts around the world who can help you to enhance your learning. Remember the fellowship triangle—training, mentors, and travel? Engaging with that triangle is something that never ends in your career!

MY-FELLOWSHIP's Growth Journey

Just as we, consulting physicians, are always seeking to grow and develop our skills, abilities, and connections with others, MY-FELLOWSHIP seeks to grow and expand its offerings.

As someone who came from Egypt and moved to Switzerland, where I currently work at the University Hospital of Basel, I had to learn German from scratch and work harder than most to build my medical career. Essentially, through lots of hard work, persistence, great mentors and perhaps even luck, I beat the odds. This is also the reason I founded the MY-FELLOWSHIP platform. MY-FELLOWSHIP was launched in collaboration with the VSAO-Basel (Association of Swiss Residents and Consultants) to provide all individuals in the medical field equal opportunity to access knowledge through fellowships and make pivotal connections by linking up information from potential fellows, past fellows, institutions, and sponsors, all of which have previously existed on separate planes and without structure. Which, in turn, made international fellowships and observerships so difficult to pursue. But not any longer!

We expect within one year to reach 1,000 subscribers on MY-FELLOWSHIP and within three years to reach 5,000 subscribers. All of these subscibers can share their fellowship or observership experiences in different medical specialties and subspecialties. Once we get sponsors, we can develop more features on the platform. In MY-FELLOWSHIP's future, we see it as the number one platform for fellowships worldwide.

As MY-FELLOWSHIP is a community-supported project, there are many different ways to contribute. If you are looking for a fellowship, you can join the platform. If you are a previous fellow, you can give feedback about the fellowship you did. If you are a fellowship provider, you can add your fellowship to that platform. Also, we welcome donations in any kind—credit card, PayPal, wire transfers—it's all available online. We urge you to support this project. Please spread the word and tell others that MY-FELLOWSHIP exists as well.

Over time, with support from the global medical community, I envision that MY-FELLOWSHIP will grow to become more than just a platform connecting individuals to streamline fellowship application processes. MY-FELLOWSHIP will evolve into a centralized hub of medical knowledge for all. Our goal is not just to make a resounding impact in the lives of doctors/researchers, but to ultimately and exponentially increase the quality of patient care.

If you would like to know more about how MY-FELLOWSHIP can help your medical career or what you can do to contribute, please visit us at www.myfellowship.com.

Never forget—the sky is the limit, it's only the beginning!

All revenue generated from this book will be donated to the community platform: www.myfellowship.com

www.ingramcontent.com/pod-product-compliance
Lightning Source LLC
Chambersburg PA
CBHW071012200526
45171CB00007B/73